Anatomy &
Physiology

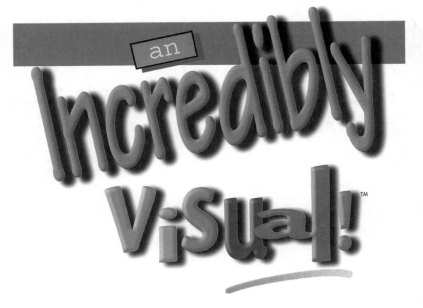

an

Pocket Guide

 Wolters Kluwer | Lippincott Williams & Wilkins
Health

Philadelphia · Baltimore · New York · London
Buenos Aires · Hong Kong · Sydney · Tokyo

Staff

Executive Publisher
Judith A. Schilling McCann, RN, MSN

Clinical Director
Joan M. Robinson, RN, MSN

Art Director
Elaine Kasmer

Clinical Project Manager
Kathryn Henry, RN, BSN, CCRC

Editors
Gale Thompson, Diane Labus

Clinical Editors
Jennifer Meyering, RN, BSN, MS, CCRN
Lisa Morris Bonsall, RN, MSN, CRNP

Illustrator
Bot Roda

Design Assistant
Kate Zulak

Associate Manufacturing Manager
Beth J. Welsh

Editorial Assistants
Karen J. Kirk, Jeri O'Shea, Linda K. Ruhf

The clinical treatments described and recommended in this publication are based on research and consultation with nursing, medical, and legal authorities. To the best of our knowledge, these procedures reflect currently accepted practice. Nevertheless, they can't be considered absolute and universal recommendations. For individual applications, all recommendations must be considered in light of the patient's clinical condition and, before administration of new or infrequently used drugs, in light of the latest package-insert information. The authors and publisher disclaim any responsibility for any adverse effects resulting from the suggested procedures, from any undetected errors, or from the reader's misunderstanding of the text.

Printed in China

A&PIVPG-010209

CONTENTS

Margaret T. Bowers, RN, MSN, FNP-BC
Assistant Clinical Professor and Nurse Practitioner
Duke University School of Nursing
Durham, N.C.

Cheryl L. Brady, RN, MSN
Assistant Professor of Nursing
Kent State University
Salem, Ohio

Kim Cooper, RN, MSN
Nursing Department Chair
Ivy Tech Community College
Terre Haute, Ind.

Shelba Durston, RN, MSN, CCRN
Nursing Instructor
San Joaquin Delta College
Stockton, Calif.

Ann S. McQueen, MSN, CRNP, RNC
Family Nurse Practitioner
HealthLink Medical Center
Southampton, Pa.

Dana Reeves, RN, MSN
Assistant Professor
University of Arkansas
Fort Smith

Roseann Regan, PhD, APRN, BC
Assistant Professor
Gwynedd Mercy College
Gwynedd, Pa.
Thomas Jefferson University
Philadelphia

Elizabeth (Libby) Richards, RN, MSN, CHES
Clinical Assistant Professor
Purdue University
West Lafayette, Ind.

Maria Elsa Rodriguez, RN, MSN, CNS
Assistant Professor of Nursing
San Diego City Community College

Elizabeth Simmons-Rowland, RN, MSN, CNS, FNE
Assistant Professor, School of Nursing
Western Carolina University
Cullowhee, N.C.

Allison J. Terry, RN, PhD, MSN
Director, Center for Nursing
Alabama Board of Nursing
Montgomery

Brigitte K. Thiele, RN, BSN
Nurse Education Consultant
Bloomfield, Mo.

Robin R. Wilkerson, RN, PhD
Professor and Director of North Mississippi
Campuses School of Nursing
University of Mississippi Medical Center
Jackson

1

The human body

I'm so excited! We're setting out to explore the structures and functions of the magnificent human body. With so many regions and dark and mysterious cavities, we're bound to dig up a few new interesting facts—and maybe even an antiquity or two. Why not tag along? I think there's room for one more!

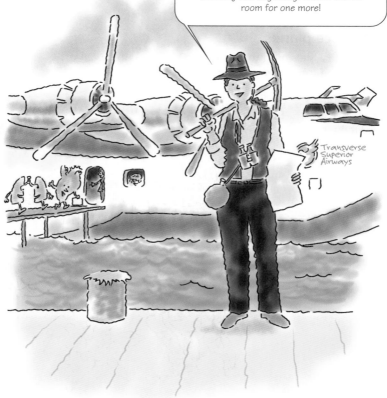

Anatomic terms

- Describe directions within the body
- Describe the body's planes, cavities, and regions

Directional terms

Generally grouped in pairs of opposites:
- *Superior* (above); *inferior* (below)
- *Anterior* or *ventral* (toward the front of the body); *posterior* or *dorsal* (toward the back of the body)
- *Medial* (toward the body's midline); *lateral* (away from the body's midline)
- *Proximal* (closest to the point of origin or the trunk); *distal* (farthest from the point of origin or the trunk)
- *Superficial* (toward or at the body surface); *deep* (farthest from the body surface)

Reference planes

- Imaginary lines used to section the body and its organs
- Consist of four major planes:
  - Median sagittal
  - Frontal
  - Transverse
  - Oblique

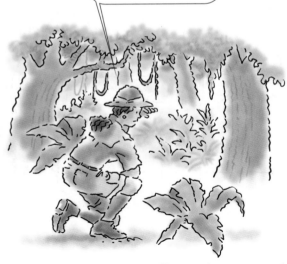

If you don't know directional terms, you won't be able to navigate the body very well.

(Text continues on page 4.)

Directional terms

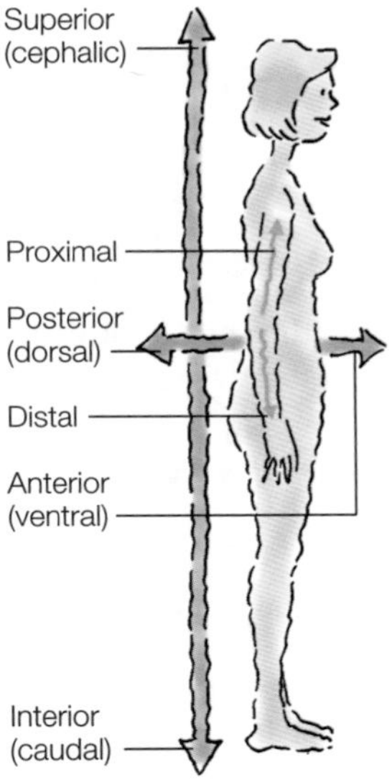

Superior
(cephalic)

Proximal

Posterior
(dorsal)

Distal

Anterior
(ventral)

Interior
(caudal)

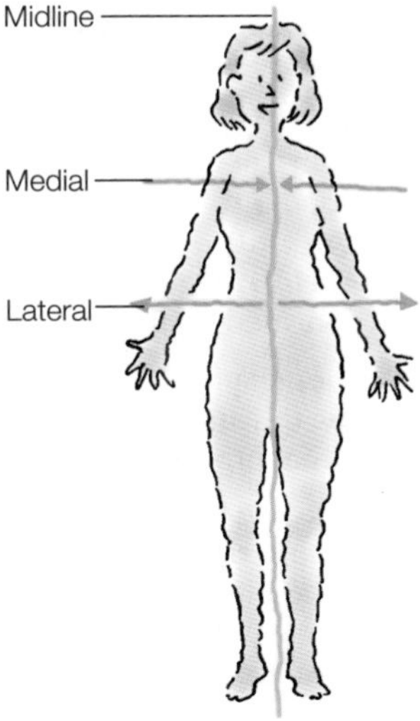

Midline

Medial

Lateral

Reference planes

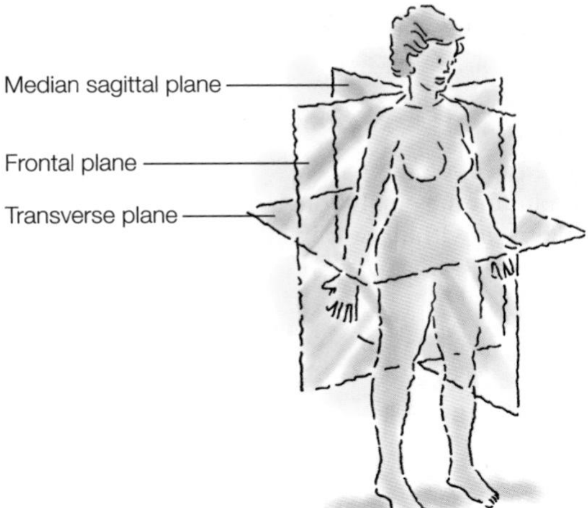

Median sagittal plane

Frontal plane

Transverse plane

Anatomic terms (continued)
Body cavities
- Spaces within the body containing internal organs
- Two major closed cavities are the *dorsal* and *ventral* cavities

Dorsal cavity
- Located in the posterior region of the body
- Subdivided into two cavities:
  - The *cranial cavity* (also called the *calvaria*): encases the brain
  - The *vertebral cavity* (also called the *spinal cavity* or *vertebral canal*): formed by the vertebrae and encloses the spinal cord

Ventral cavity
- Occupies the anterior region of the trunk
- Subdivided into the *thoracic* and *abdominopelvic* cavities

Thoracic cavity
- Located superior to the abdominopelvic cavity
- Subdivided into two *pleural cavities* (each contains a lung) and the *mediastinum* (which contains the heart, large vessels of the heart, trachea, esophagus, thymus, lymph nodes, and other blood vessels and nerves)

Abdominopelvic cavity
- Divided into the *abdominal cavity* and the *pelvic cavity*
- Abdominal cavity: contains the stomach, intestines, spleen, liver, and other organs
- Pelvic cavity: contains the bladder, some of the reproductive organs, and the rectum

Other cavities
- *Oral*: the mouth
- *Orbital*: house the eyes
- *Middle ear*: contain the small bones of the middle ear
- *Synovial*: enclosed within the capsules surrounding freely movable joints

(Text continues on page 6.)

Locating body cavities

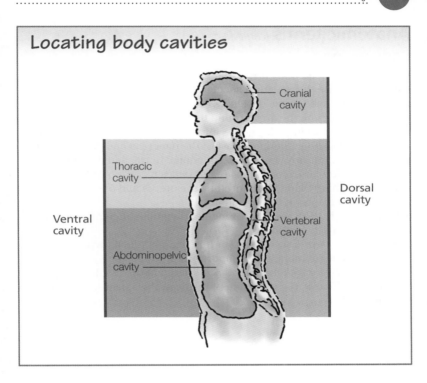

Cranial cavity

Thoracic cavity

Dorsal cavity

Ventral cavity

Vertebral cavity

Abdominopelvic cavity

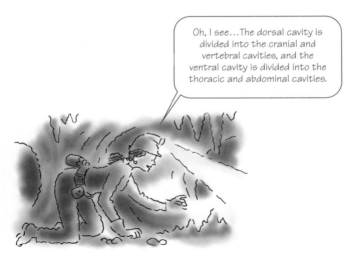

Oh, I see...The dorsal cavity is divided into the cranial and vertebral cavities, and the ventral cavity is divided into the thoracic and abdominal cavities.

Anatomic terms *(continued)*

Body regions

- Used to designate body areas that have special nerves or vascular supplies or those that perform special functions
- Most widely used terms designate sections of the abdomen
- *Umbilical region*: the area around the umbilicus; includes sections of the small and large intestines, inferior vena cava, and abdominal aorta
- *Epigastric region*: contains most of the pancreas and portions of the stomach, liver, inferior vena cava, abdominal aorta, and duodenum
- *Hypogastric region* (or pubic area): houses a portion of the sigmoid colon, the urinary bladder and ureters, the uterus and ovaries (in females), and portions of the small intestine
- Right and left *iliac regions* (or inguinal regions): include portions of the small and large intestines
- Right and left *lumbar regions* (or loin regions): include portions of the small and large intestines and portions of the kidneys
- Right and left *hypochondriac regions*: contain the diaphragm, portions of the kidneys, the right side of the liver, the spleen, and part of the pancreas

Identifying abdominal regions

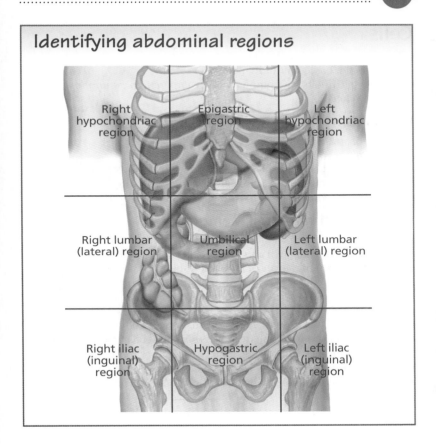

Cells

- Make up the body's structure
- Serve as the basic unit of living matter
- Consist of three basic components: *protoplasm, plasma membrane,* and the *nucleus*

Protoplasm

- A viscous, translucent, watery material
- The primary component of plant and animal cells
- Contains a large percentage of water, inorganic ions (such as potassium, calcium, magnesium, and sodium), and naturally occurring organic compounds (such as proteins, lipids, and carbohydrates)

Plasma membrane (cell membrane)

- Acts as the cell's external boundary by separating it from other cells and from the external environment
- Consists of a double layer of phospholipids with protein molecules

Nucleus

- The cell's "mission control"
- Plays a role in cell growth, metabolism, and reproduction
- A nucleus may contain one or more *nucleoli*—a dark-staining structure that synthesizes ribonucleic acid (RNA)
- The nucleus also contains chromosomes that control cellular activity and direct protein synthesis through ribosomes in the cytoplasm

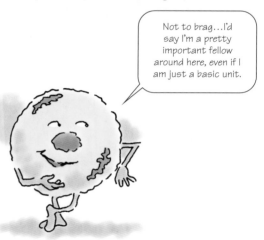

Not to brag...I'd say I'm a pretty important fellow around here, even if I am just a basic unit.

Inside the cell

Cytoplasm (protoplasm that
surrounds the nucleus)

Cell membrane
(encloses the cell)

Mitochondrion
(production site of
adenosine triphosphate—
cellular energy)

Centriole
(takes part in cell division)

Endoplasmic reticulum
(transports protein and lipid
components)

Ribosomes
(sites for protein synthesis)

Golgi complex (processes
and packages protein)

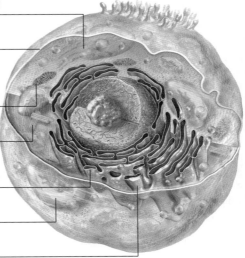

Microvilli (increase
surface size of the cell)

Nucleus (brain of the cell)

Nucleolus (site of
ribosomal RNA synthesis)

Ribonucleic acid
(transfers genetic
information to ribosomes)

Chromatin (complex of
DNA, RNA, and protein
that makes up
chromosomes)

Lysosome (contains
digestive enzymes)

DNA and RNA

- New tissue growth, and the repair of damaged tissue, depends on protein synthesis
- This process involves DNA and RNA

DNA

- Carries genetic information and provides the blueprint for protein synthesis
- Consists of a basic structural unit called a *nucleotide* (which consists of a phosphate group linked to a five-carbon sugar, *deoxyribose*, and joined to a nitrogen-containing compound called a *base*)
- Four different DNA bases exist: adenine (A); guanine (G); thymine (T); and cytosine (C)
- Adenine bonds only with thymine; guanine bonds only with cytosine

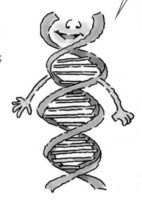

I'm the double-stranded nucleic acid that carries the hereditary information and the blueprint for protein synthesis. You can't get along without me.

RNA

- Consists of nucleotide chains that differ slightly from the nucleotide chains found in DNA
- Transfers genetic information to the *ribosomes*, where protein synthesis occurs
- Types of RNA involved in the transfer are ribosomal, messenger, and transfer RNA

Types of RNA

Types of RNA

Ribosomal RNA
- Used to make ribosomes in the endoplasmic reticulum of the cytoplasm, where the cell produces proteins

Messenger RNA
- Directs the arrangement of amino acids to make proteins at the ribosomes
- Contains a single strand of nucleotides that's complementary to a segment of the DNA chain that contains instructions for protein synthesis
- Contains chains that pass from the nucleus into the cytoplasm, where they attach to ribosomes

Transfer RNA
- Consists of short nucleotide chains, each of which is specific for an individual amino acid
- Transfers the genetic code from messenger RNA for the production of a specific amino acid

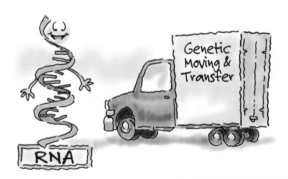

Genetic Moving & Transfer

RNA

Cell reproduction

- Cells must reproduce or die
- Cells reproduce (replicate) through division
- Before a cell divides, its chromosomes are duplicated
- During cell division, the double helix separates into two DNA chains, each serving as a template for a new chain
- Individual DNA nucleotides are linked into new strands with bases complementary to those in the original
- Two identical double helices are formed, each containing one of the original strands and a newly formed complementary strand
- These double helices are duplicates of the original DNA chain
- Cells use the processes of *mitosis* or *meiosis* to replicate

(Text continues on page 14.)

Cell division

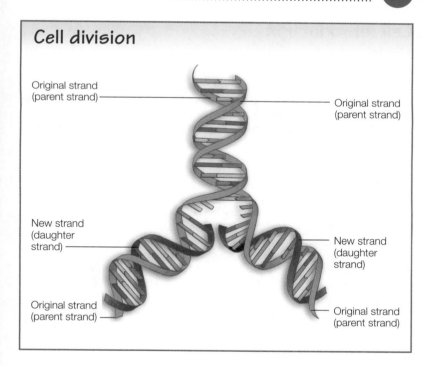

Original strand (parent strand)

Original strand (parent strand)

New strand (daughter strand)

New strand (daughter strand)

Original strand (parent strand)

Original strand (parent strand)

Cell reproduction *(continued)*

Mitosis

● Involves the equal division of material in the nucleus (*karyokinesis*) followed by division of the cell body (*cytokinesis*)

● Occurs in five phases: an inactive phase (*interphase*) and four active phases (*prophase, metaphase, anaphase,* and *telophase*)

● Results in two daughter cells (exact duplicates), each containing 23 pairs of chromosomes—or 46 individual chromosomes; this number is the *diploid number*

Meiosis

● Reserved for gametes (ova and spermatozoa)

● Intermixes genetic material between homologous chromosomes, producing four daughter cells, each with the *haploid number* of chromosomes (23, or half of the 46)

● Has two divisions separated by a resting phase

● The first division has six phases; it begins with one parent cell and ends with two daughter cells—each containing the haploid (23) number of chromosomes

● The second division resembles mitosis and has four phases; it starts with two new daughter cells (each containing the haploid number of chromosomes) and ends with four new haploid cells

The active phases of mitosis

1 Prophase

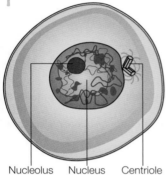

Nucleolus   Nucleus   Centriole

2 Metaphase

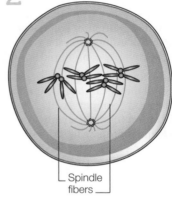

Spindle fibers

3 Anaphase

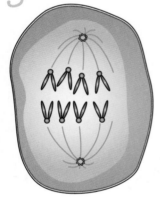

4 Telophase

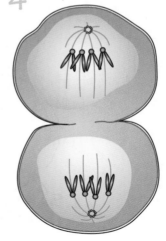

Movement within cells

- Cellular function depends on energy generation and transportation of substances within and among cells
- Transport methods may be passive or active

Passive transport

- Requires no energy
- Includes *diffusion* and *osmosis*

Diffusion

- Solutes move from an area of higher to lower concentration until an equal distribution of solutes occurs
- Factors influencing the rate of diffusion include concentration gradient, particle size, and lipid solubility

Osmosis

- Fluid moves across a membrane from an area of lower solute concentration (comparatively *more* fluid) into an area of higher solute concentration (comparatively *less* fluid)
- Osmosis stops when the solute concentration on each side of the membrane becomes equalized

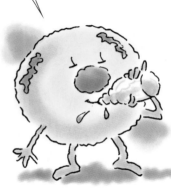

I find that a quenching glass of water and a few minutes of peace and quiet are sometimes all I need to absorb a difficult concept such as osmosis.

(Text continues on page 18.)

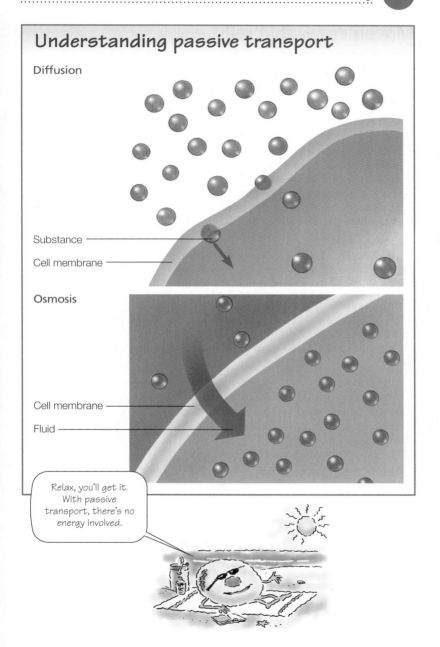

Understanding passive transport

Diffusion

Substance

Cell membrane

Osmosis

Cell membrane

Fluid

Relax, you'll get it. With passive transport, there's no energy involved.

Movement within cells *(continued)*

Active transport

- Requires energy
- Usually moves a substance across the cell membrane against the concentration gradient (from an area of lower to higher concentration)
- Processes include *sodium-potassium pump*, *pinocytosis*, *endocytosis*, and *filtration*

Sodium-potassium pump

- Moves sodium from inside the cell to outside, where the sodium concentration is greater; moves potassium from outside the cell to inside, where the potassium concentration is greater
- The energy required for this movement provided by adenosine triphosphate (ATP)

Pinocytosis

- Tiny vacuoles take droplets of fluid containing dissolved substances into the cell
- The cell uses the engulfed fluid

Endocytosis

- The cell surrounds a substance with part of its cell membrane to engulf it
- This part separates to form a *vacuole* (cavity) that moves to the cell's interior

Filtration

- Pressure (provided by capillary blood) forces fluid and dissolved particles through the cell membrane and into the interstitial fluid
- The rate of filtration varies according to the pressure

> Active transport takes some effort to move particles from one side of the membrane across to the other side. But it's like they say, "No pain, no gain."

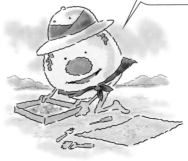

Understanding active transport

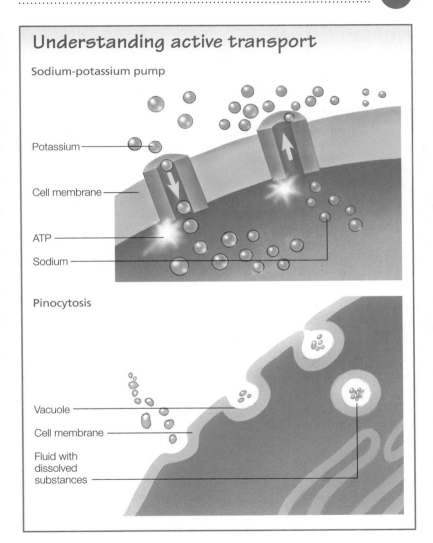

Sodium-potassium pump

Potassium —

Cell membrane —

ATP —

Sodium —

Pinocytosis

Vacuole —

Cell membrane —

Fluid with
dissolved
substances —

Human tissue

- Defined as groups of cells that perform the same general function
- Consist of four basic types: *epithelial, connective, muscle*, and *nervous*

Epithelial tissue

- A continuous cellular sheet that covers the body's surface, lines body cavities, and forms certain glands
- Classified by the number of cell layers and the shape of the surface cells
    - *Simple*: one layer
    - *Stratified*: multilayered
    - *Pseudostratified*: one layer, but appears multilayered
    - *Squamous*: contains flat surface cells
    - *Columnar*: contains tall, cylindrical surface cells
    - *Cuboidal*: contains cube-shaped surface cells

(Text continues on page 22.)

Types of epithelial tissue

Type	Function	
Simple squamous	Lines blood vessels, lymph nodes, and the alveoli of the lungs	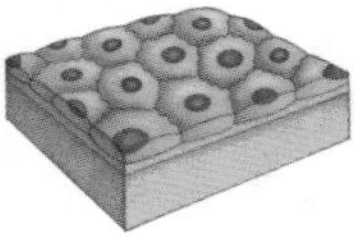
Simple columnar epithelium	Lines the intestines	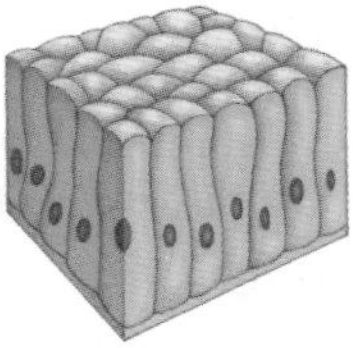
Simple cuboidal epithelium	Found on the surface of the ovary and the thyroid	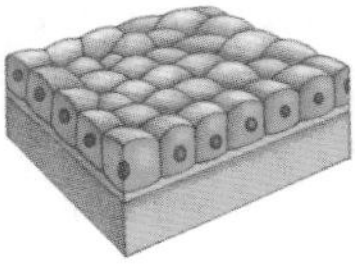
Stratified squamous epithelium	Makes up the epidermis of the skin	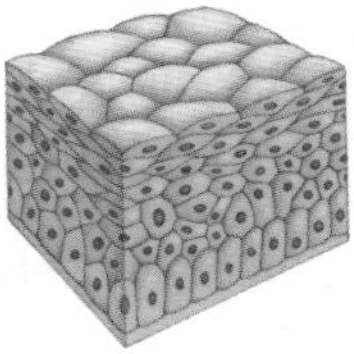
Stratified columnar epithelium	Found in the ducts	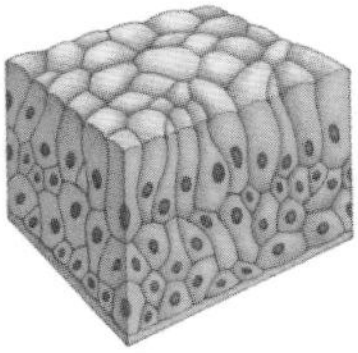
Pseudostratified columnar epithelium	Form the lining of the respiratory tract	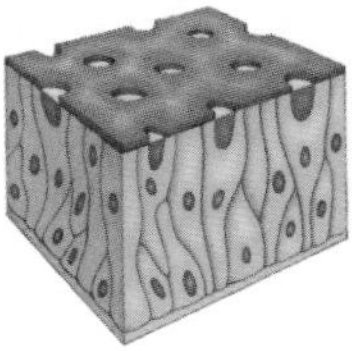

Human tissue *(continued)*

Connective tissue

- Includes bone, cartilage, and adipose (fatty) tissue
- Binds together and supports body structures
- Classified as *loose* or *dense*

Loose (areolar)

- Has large spaces that separate the fibers and cells
- Contains a lot of intercellular fluid
- *Adipose tissue* (fat) is a specialized type of loose connective tissue
  - Insulates the body to conserve body heat
  - Cushions internal organs
  - Stores excess food and reserve supplies of energy

Dense

- Provides structural support
- Has greater fiber concentration
- Is further subdivided into dense regular and dense irregular connective tissue

Dense regular

- Consists of tightly packed fibers arranged in a consistent pattern
- Includes tendons, ligaments, and *aponeuroses* (flat fibrous sheets that attach muscles to bones or other tissues)

Dense irregular

- Has tightly packed fibers arranged in an inconsistent pattern
- Found in the dermis, submucosa of the GI tract, fibrous capsules, and fasciae

(Text continues on page 24.)

Adipose tissue

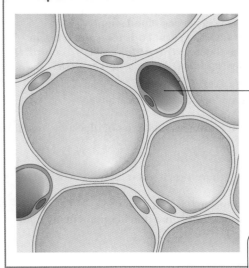

In this tissue, a single lipid (fat) droplet occupies most of each cell.

Adipose tissue is a special connective tissue that acts as an insulator to conserve body heat, as a cushion for internal organs, and as a storage depot for excess food and energy.

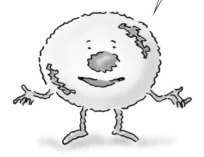

Human tissue *(continued)*

Muscle tissue

- Consists of muscle cells with a generous blood supply
- Muscle cells measure up to several centimeters long and have an elongated shape that enhances their *contractility* (ability to contract)
- Consists of three basic types: *striated, cardiac,* and *smooth*

Striated

- Gets its name from its striped, or striated, appearance
- Contracts voluntarily
- Found in muscles that guard entrances and exits of digestive, respiratory, and urinary tracts

Cardiac

- Composed of striated tissue (therefore, it's sometimes classified as striated)
- Differs from other striated muscle tissue in two ways
  - Its fibers are separate cellular units that don't contain many nuclei
- Found in the heart

Smooth

- Consists of long, spindle-shaped cells and lacks the striped pattern of striated tissue
- Isn't under voluntary control (its activity is stimulated by the autonomic nervous system)
- Lines many internal organs and other structures

(Text continues on page 26.)

Types of muscle tissue

Striated muscle

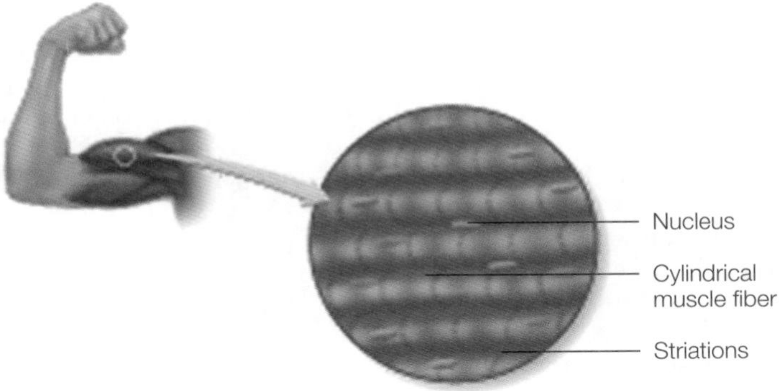

Nucleus

Cylindrical muscle fiber

Striations

Cardiac muscle

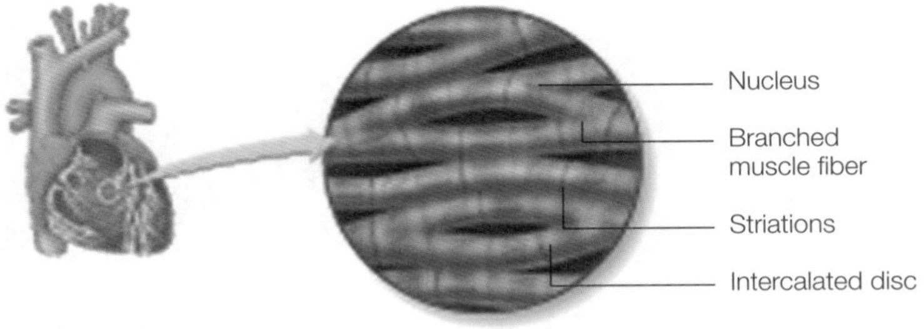

Nucleus

Branched muscle fiber

Striations

Intercalated disc

Smooth muscle

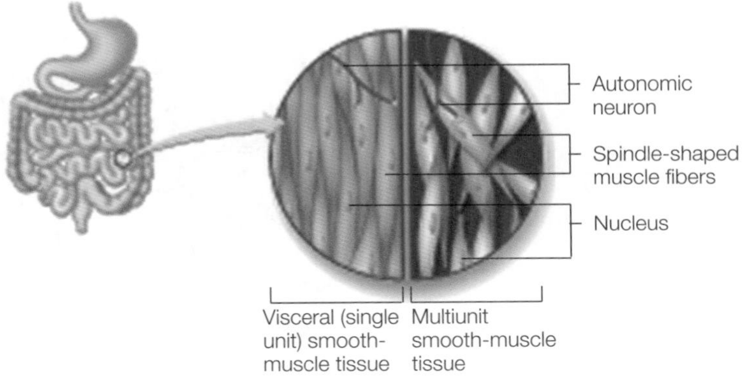

Autonomic neuron

Spindle-shaped muscle fibers

Nucleus

Visceral (single unit) smooth-muscle tissue

Multiunit smooth-muscle tissue

Human tissue *(continued)*

Nervous tissue

- Main function is communication
- Has two primary properties
  - *Irritability*: the capacity to react to various physical and chemical agents
  - *Conductivity*: the ability to transmit the reaction from one point to another
- Contains *neurons* (highly specialized cells that generate and conduct nerve impulses)
  - Typically consists of a cell body with cytoplasmic extensions—numerous *dendrites* on one pole and a single *axon* on the opposite pole
  - Extensions allow the neuron to conduct impulses over long distances
- Supporting structure formed by *neuroglia*
  - Insulate and protect neurons
  - Found only in the central nervous system

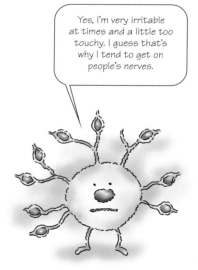

Yes, I'm very irritable at times and a little too touchy. I guess that's why I tend to get on people's nerves.

The neuron

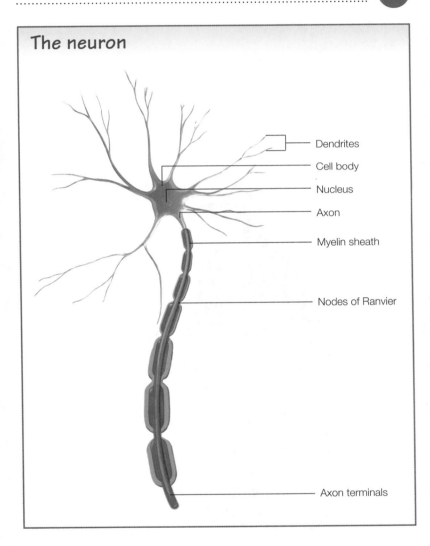

Dendrites

Cell body

Nucleus

Axon

Myelin sheath

Nodes of Ranvier

Axon terminals

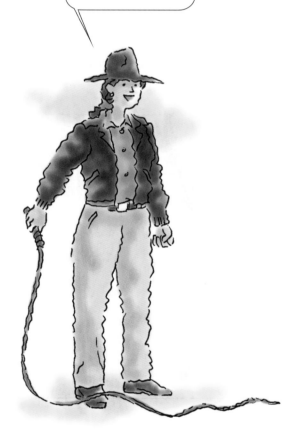

2

Genetics

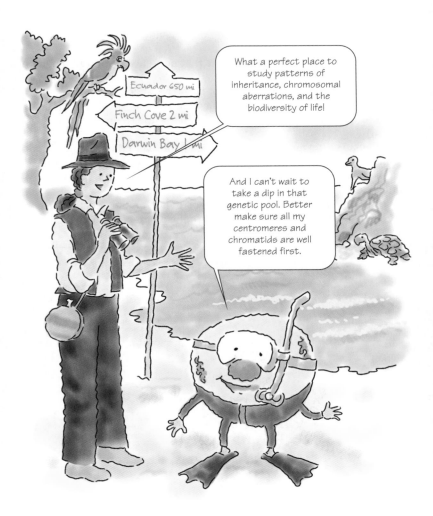

Genetics basics

● Genetics is defined as the study of heredity: the passing of traits from biological parents to their children
● Genetic information is carried in *genes*, which are strung together on the *deoxyribonucleic acid* (DNA) double helix to form chromosomes

Chromosomes

● Carried within the nucleus of each germ cell
● Each chromosome contains a strand of genetic material called *DNA*
  – DNA is a long molecule made up of thousands of segments called *genes*
  – Genes carry the code for proteins that influence each trait a person inherits
● Chromosomes exist in pairs except in the germ cells
  – A human ovum contains 23 chromosomes; a sperm also contains 23 chromosomes (each similar in size and shape to those in the ovum)
  – When an ovum and a sperm unite, the corresponding chromosomes pair up
  – The result is a fertilized cell with 46 chromosomes (23 pairs) in its nucleus
● Of the 23 pairs of chromosomes in each living human cell, the two sex chromosomes of the 23rd pair determine a person's gender
● The other 22 pairs are called *autosomes*

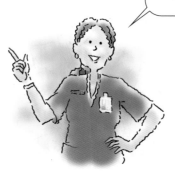

Remember, each germ cell (that's an ovum or a sperm) contains 23 chromosomes. When an ovum and a sperm unite, they form a fertilized cell with a full complement of 46 chromosomes in its nucleus.

(Text continues on page 32.)

A close look at a chromosome

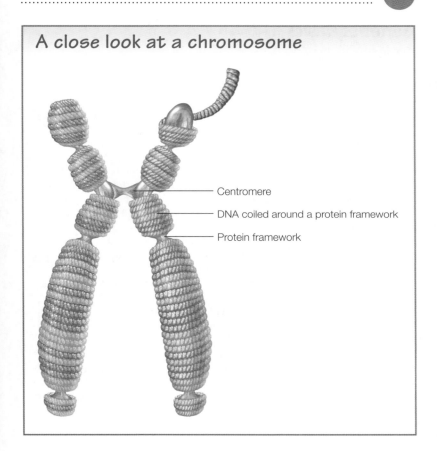

Centromere

DNA coiled around a protein framework

Protein framework

Genetics basics *(continued)*

Genes

- Segments of a DNA chain
  - Arranged in sequence on a chromosome
  - Sequence determines the properties of an organism
- *Gene locus*: the location of a specific gene on a chromosome
  - Gene locus doesn't vary from person to person
  - This allows genes in an ovum to join the corresponding genes from a sperm at fertilization
  - Genetic information stored at a locus of a gene determines the genetic constitution—or genotype—of a person; the detectable, outward manifestation of a genotype is called the phenotype
- *Genome*: one complete set of chromosomes, containing all the genetic information for one person
- Each parent contributes one set of chromosomes (and therefore one set of genes) to their offspring; therefore, every offspring has two genes for every locus on the autosomal chromosomes
- Some characteristics, or traits, are determined by one gene that may have many variants
  - Variations of the same gene are called *alleles*
  - A person who has identical alleles on each chromosome is *homozygous* for that trait
  - If the alleles are different, they're said to be *heterozygous*
- Other traits—called *polygenic traits*—require the interaction of more than one gene
- *Gene expression*: the effect that a gene has on cell structure or function
- Gene expression can vary with the gene and may be dominant, recessive, codominant, or sex-linked

(Text continues on page 34.)

How genes express themselves

Dominant genes	Recessive genes	Codominant genes	Sex-linked genes
• If genes could speak, dominant genes would be loud and garrulous, dominating every conversation!	• Unlike dominant genes, recessive genes prefer to hide their light under a bushel basket.	• Firm believers in equality, codominant genes (such as the genes that direct specific types of hemoglobin synthesis in red blood cells) allow expression of both alleles.	• Sex-linked genes are carried on sex chromosomes.
• Dominant genes (such as the one for dark hair) can be expressed and transmitted to the offspring even if only one parent possesses the gene.	• A recessive gene (such as the one for blond hair) is expressed only when both parents transmit it to the offspring.		• Almost all appear on the X chromosome and are recessive.
			• In the male, sex-linked genes behave like dominant genes because no second X chromosome exists.

Genetics basics (continued)

Autosomal inheritance

- On autosomal chromosomes, one allele may exert more influence in determining a specific trait; this is called the *dominant gene*
- Offspring express the trait of a dominant allele if both, or only one, chromosome in a pair carries it
- The less influential allele is called the *recessive gene*
- For a recessive allele to be expressed, both chromosomes must carry recessive versions of the alleles

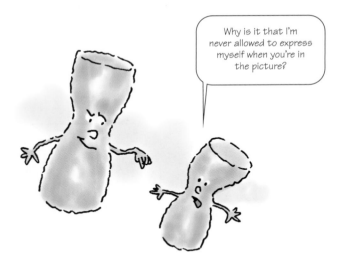

(Text continues on page 36.)

Understanding autosomal inheritance

Autosomal dominant inheritance

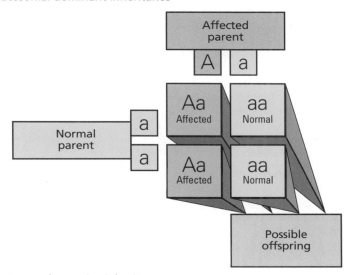

Autosomal recessive inheritance

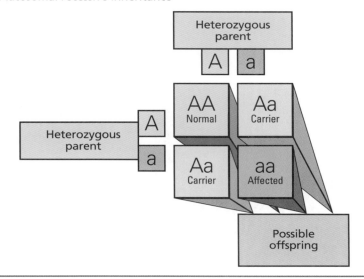

Genetics basics (continued)
Sex-linked inheritance

- The X and Y chromosomes are the sex chromosomes
- The X chromosome is much larger than the Y
- Males (who have XY chromosomes) have less genetic material than females (who have XX chromosomes)
- Therefore, they have only one copy of most genes on the X chromosome
- Because male offspring receive a Y chromosome, fathers transmit X-linked genes only to their daughters
- Inheritance of those genes is called *X-linked*, or *sex-linked, inheritance*
- A woman transmits one copy of each X-linked gene to each of her children, male or female

X-linked dominant inheritance
- When the father is affected, only his daughters have the abnormal gene
- When the mother is affected, both male and female offspring may be affected

(Text continues on page 38.)

Understanding X-linked dominant inheritance

This diagram shows the possible off-spring of a normal parent and a parent with an X-linked dominant gene on the X chromosome (shown by a solid dot).

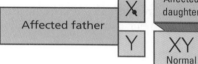

Normal mother

X X

Affected father

X

Y

XX Affected daughter

XX Affected daughter

XY Normal son

XY Normal son

Possible offspring

Affected mother

X X

Normal father

X

Y

XX Affected daughter

XX Normal daughter

XY Affected son

XY Normal son

Possible offspring

Genetics basics *(continued)*

Sex-linked inheritance *(continued)*

X-linked recessive inheritance

● All female offspring of an affected male will be carriers
● The son of a female carrier may inherit a recessive gene on the X chromosome and be affected by the disease

Multifactorial inheritance

● Reflects the interaction of at least two genes and the influence of environmental factors
　– Height is a classic example
　– The parents' height as well as nutritional patterns, health care, and other environmental factors influence an offspring's height development
● Some diseases also have genetic predispositions for multifactorial inheritance (a disease might be expressed only under certain environmental conditions)

Factors contributing to multifactorial inheritance

● Maternal age
● Use of drugs, alcohol, or hormones by either parent
● Maternal or paternal exposure to radiation
● Maternal infection during pregnancy or existing diseases in the mother
● Nutritional factors
● General maternal or paternal health
● High altitude
● Maternal smoking
● Maternal-fetal blood incompatibility
● Inadequate prenatal care

Understanding X-linked recessive inheritance

This diagram shows the possible off-spring of a normal parent and a parent with a recessive gene on the X chromosome (shown by an open dot).

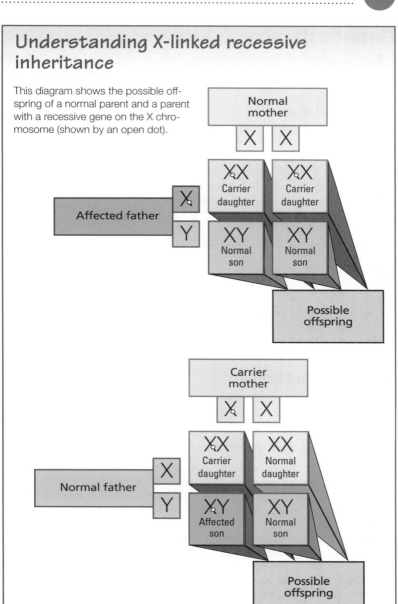

Genetic defects

- Defects that result from changes to genes or chromosomes
- Categorized as either *autosomal disorders*, *sex-linked disorders*, or *multifactorial disorders*

Autosomal disorders

- Disorders in which an error occurs at a single gene site on the DNA strand
- Causes most hereditary disorders
- *Autosomal dominant transmission* involves the transmission of an abnormal gene that's dominant; *autosomal recessive inheritance* involves transmission of an abnormal recessive gene

Sex-linked disorders

- Disorders caused by genes located on the sex chromosomes
- Most are controlled by genes on the X chromosome, usually as recessive traits
- Because males have only one X chromosome, a single X-linked recessive gene can cause disease to be exhibited in a male
- Females receive two X chromosomes, so they may be homozygous for a disease allele (and exhibit the disease), homozygous for a normal allele (and neither have nor carry the disease), or heterozygous (carry, but not exhibit, the disease)

Multifactorial disorders

- May result from both genetic and environmental factors
- Can result from a less-than-optimum expression of many different genes, not from a specific error

Chromosome defects

- Aberrations in chromosome structure or number cause a class of disorders called *congenital anomalies*, or *birth defects*
- Genetic aberrations include the loss, addition, or rearrangement of genetic material
- *Translocation* occurs when chromosomes split apart and rejoin in an abnormal arrangement; children of parents with translocated chromosomes may have serious genetic defects, such as monosomies or trisomies
- During meiosis and mitosis, chromosomes normally separate in a process called *disjunction*
- Failure to separate (*nondisjunction*) causes an unequal distribution of chromosomes between the two resulting cells

Chromosomal disjunction and nondisjunction

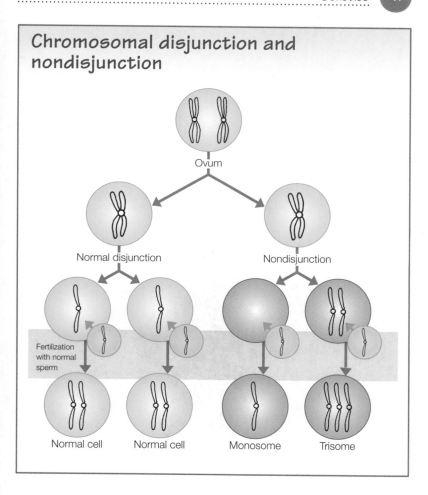

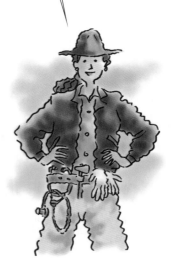

Chemical organization

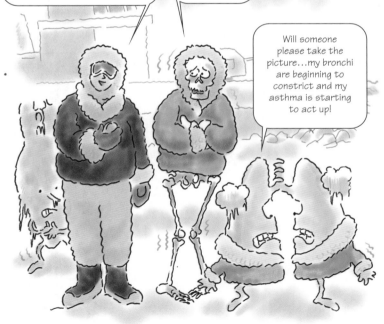

Body chemistry

- Every cell contains thousands of different chemicals that constantly interact with one another
- Types of body tissues are differentiated based on chemical composition
- The blueprints of heredity (deoxyribonucleic acid [DNA] and ribonucleic acid [RNA]) are encoded in chemical form
- *Matter*: anything (solid, liquid, or gas) that has mass and occupies space
- *Energy*: the capacity to do work (to put mass into motion)
  - *Potential energy*: stored energy
  - *Kinetic energy*: the energy of motion
  - Types of energy include chemical, electrical, and radiant

Chemical composition

- *Element*: matter that can't be broken down into simpler substances by normal chemical reactions
- All forms of matter are composed of chemical elements
- Each chemical element in the periodic table has a chemical symbol
- Carbon, hydrogen, nitrogen, and oxygen account for 96% of the body's total weight
- Calcium and phosphorus account for another 2.5%

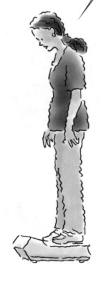

When you think of body weight in terms of carbon, hydrogen, nitrogen, and oxygen, it doesn't seem that bad. But it all adds up fast, doesn't it?

What's a body made of?

- Oxygen 65%
- Carbon 18.5%
- Hydrogen 9.5%
- Nitrogen 3.3%
- Calcium 1.5%
- Phosphorus 1%
- Potassium 0.4%
- Sulfur 0.3%
- Chlorine 0.2%
- Sodium 0.2%
- Magnesium 0.1%
- Iron 0.004%
- Iodine 0.00004%
- Trace elements
  - Silicon
  - Fluorine
  - Copper
  - Manganese
  - Zinc
  - Selenium
  - Cobalt
  - Molybdenum
  - Boron

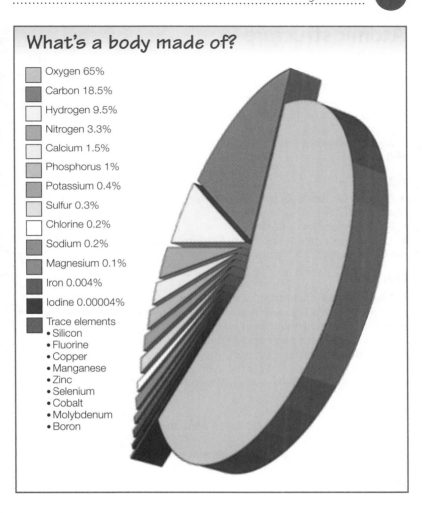

Atomic structure

- *Atom*: the smallest unit of matter that can take part in a chemical reaction
- Each atom has a dense central core called a *nucleus*
- *Molecule*: a combination of two or more atoms of the same element
- *Compound*: a combination of two or more atoms that are different elements
- Atoms consist of three basic subatomic particles: *protons*, *neutrons*, and *electrons*

Protons

- *Protons* (p^+): closely packed, positively charged particles in the atom's nucleus
- Each element has a distinct number of protons
- An element's number of protons determines its *atomic number* and positive charge

Neutrons

- *Neutrons* (n): uncharged, or neutral, particles in the atom's nucleus
- An atom's *atomic mass number* is the sum of the number of protons and neutrons in the nucleus of an atom
- *Isotope*: a form of an atom that has a different number of neutrons and, therefore, a different atomic weight
- An atom's *atomic weight* is the average of the relative weights (atomic mass numbers) of all the element's isotopes

Electrons

- *Electrons* (e^-): negatively charged particles that orbit the nucleus in electron shells
- Play a key role in chemical bonds and reactions
- The number of electrons in an atom equals the number of protons in its nucleus
- The electrons' negative charges cancel out the protons' positive charges, making atoms electrically neutral

(Text continues on page 48.)

Subatomic particles

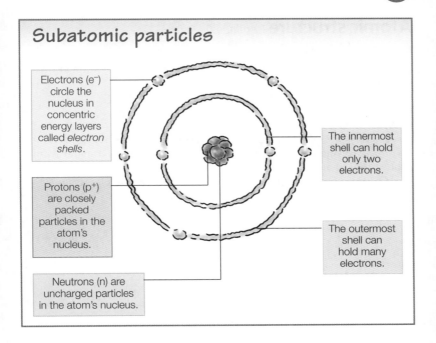

Electrons (e⁻) circle the nucleus in concentric energy layers called *electron shells*.

The innermost shell can hold only two electrons.

Protons (p⁺) are closely packed particles in the atom's nucleus.

The outermost shell can hold many electrons.

Neutrons (n) are uncharged particles in the atom's nucleus.

Atomic structure (continued)
Chemical bonds

- *Chemical bond*: a force of attraction that binds a molecule's atoms together
- Formation of a chemical bond usually requires energy
- Breakup of a chemical bond usually releases energy
- Types of chemical bonds:
  - *Hydrogen bond*: when two atoms associate with a hydrogen atom
  - *Ionic* (electrovalent) *bond*: when valence electrons transfer from one atom to another
  - *Covalent bond*: when atoms share pairs of valence electrons

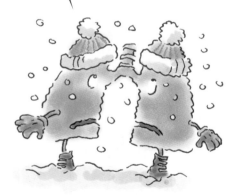

(Text continues on page 50.)

Types of chemical bonds

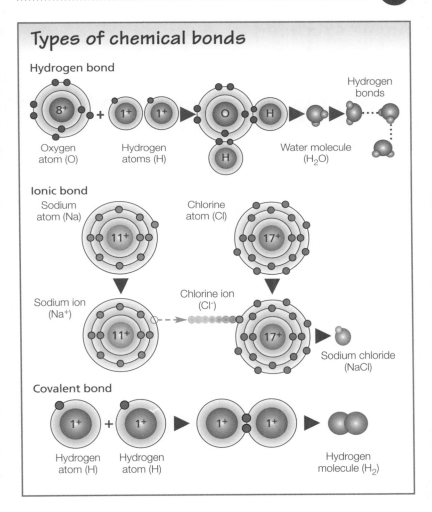

Hydrogen bond

Oxygen atom (O) + Hydrogen atoms (H) → Water molecule (H_2O)

Hydrogen bonds

Ionic bond

Sodium atom (Na)

Chlorine atom (Cl)

Sodium ion (Na^+)

Chlorine ion (Cl^-)

Sodium chloride (NaCl)

Covalent bond

Hydrogen atom (H) + Hydrogen atom (H) → Hydrogen molecule (H_2)

Atomic structure *(continued)*

Chemical reactions

- Involves unpaired electrons in the outer shells of atoms
- One of two events occurs:
  - Unpaired electrons from the outer shell of one atom transfer to the outer shell of another atom
  - One atom shares its unpaired electrons with another atom
- Energy, particle concentration, speed, and orientation determine whether a chemical reaction will occur
- Four basic types of chemical reactions: *synthesis*, *decomposition*, *exchange*, and *reversible reactions*

Four basic types of chemical reactions

- **Synthesis:** Two or more substances combine to form a new, more complex substance

$$A + B \rightarrow AB$$

- **Decomposition:** One substance breaks down into two or more simpler substances

$$AB \rightarrow A + B$$

- **Exchange:** A combination of decomposition and synthesis

$$AB + CD \rightarrow A + B + C + D \rightarrow AD + BC$$

- **Reversible:** The product may revert back to its original reactant or vice versa

$$A \rightarrow B \leftrightarrow AB$$

In a chemical reaction, unpaired electrons from one atom can be transferred to another atom's outer shell or they can be shared with the other atom.

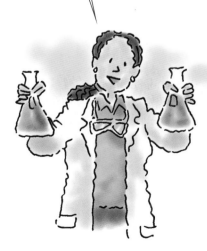

Inorganic and organic compounds

- Most biomolecules (molecules produced by living cells) form *organic compounds* (compounds containing carbon or carbon-hydrogen bonds)
- Some form *inorganic compounds* (compounds without carbon)

Inorganic compounds

- Usually small and include water and *electrolytes*—inorganic acids, bases, and salts
- Electrolytes: compounds whose molecules consist of positively charged ions (*cations*) and negatively charged ions (*anions*) that separate into ions (*ionize*) in solution
  - *Acids* ionize into hydrogen ions (H^+) and anions
  - *Bases* ionize into hydroxide ions and cations
  - *Salts* form when acids react with bases; in water, they ionize into cations and anions
- Body fluids must attain acid-base balance to maintain *homeostasis*
  - The number of hydrogen ions in a solution determines its acidity
  - The more hydrogen ions present, the more acidic the solution
  - The more hydroxide ions present, the more basic (*alkaline*) the solution

Organic compounds

- Examples include *carbohydrates*, *lipids*, *proteins*, and *nucleic acids*

Carbohydrates

- In the body, *carbohydrates* are sugars, starches, and glycogen
- Three types of carbohydrates: monosaccharides, disaccharides, and polysaccharides

Lipids

- Consist of water-insoluble biomolecules
- Major lipids: *triglycerides*, *phospholipids*, *steroids*, *lipoproteins*, and *eicosanoids*

(Text continues on page 54.)

A closer look at carbohydrates and lipids

Carbohydrate molecule

Lipid molecule

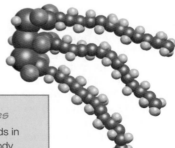

Types of lipids

Triglycerides
- Most abundant lipids in both food and the body
- Neutral fats that insulate and protect
- The body's most concentrated energy source

Lipoproteins
- Help transport lipids to various parts of the body

Sterols
- Simple lipids with no fatty acids in their molecules
- Fall into four main categories:

 Bile salts: emulsify fats during digestion and aid absorption of the fat-soluble vitamins (vitamins A, D, E, and K)

 Male and female sex hormones: responsible for sexual characteristics and reproduction

Cholesterol: a part of animal cell membranes; needed to form all other sterols

Vitamin D: helps regulate the body's calcium concentration

Phospholipids
- Major structural components of cell membranes
- Consist of one molecule of glycerol, two molecules of a fatty acid, and a phosphate group

Eicosanoids
- Prostaglandins: modify hormone responses, promote the inflammatory response, and open the airways
- Leukotrienes: play a part in allergic and inflammatory responses

Inorganic and organic compounds *(continued)*
Organic compounds *(continued)*

Proteins

- The most abundant organic compound in the body
- Composed of building blocks called *amino acids*
- Amino acids are linked together by *peptide bonds*
- Many amino acids linked together form a *polypeptide*
- One or more polypeptides form a protein
- The sequence of amino acids in a protein's polypeptide chain dictates its shape, which determines the function it may perform:
  - providing structure and protection
  - regulating processes
  - promoting muscle contraction
  - serving as an enzyme
  - transporting various substances

Nucleic acids

- Include DNA and RNA
- Both DNA and RNA are composed of nitrogenous bases, sugars, and phosphate groups

DNA

- Primary hereditary molecule
- Contains two long chains of deoxyribonucleotides coiled into a double-helix shape
- Deoxyribose and phosphate units alternate in the "backbone" of the chains
- Holding the two chains together are base pairs of adenine-thymine and guanine-cytosine

RNA

- Has a single-chain structure
- Contains ribose instead of deoxyribose and replaces the base thymine with uracil
- Transmits genetic information from the cell nucleus to the cytoplasm
- In the cytoplasm, it guides protein synthesis from amino acids

A closer look at proteins and nucleic acids

Protein molecule

Nucleic acid

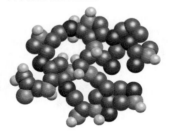

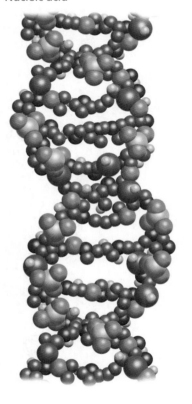

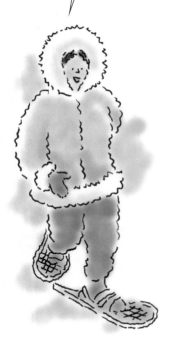

4

Integumentary system

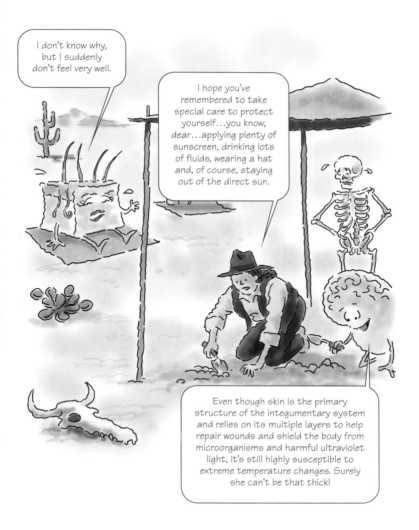

Integumentary system

- Considered to be the largest body system
- Includes the skin (*integument*) and its appendages (the hair, nails, and certain glands)
- Consists of two distinct layers—the *epidermis* and *dermis*—above a third layer of *subcutaneous tissue* (sometimes called the *hypodermis*)

Layer	Sublayers
Epidermis • Outermost layer • Varies in thickness from less than 0.1 mm (on the eyelids) to more than 1 mm (on the palms and soles) • Composed of avascular, stratified, squamous (scaly or platelike) epithelial tissue • Consists of five sublayers	Stratum corneum • Outermost layer • Consists of tightly arranged layers of cellular membranes and keratin Stratum lucidum • Lucid or clear layer • Blocks water penetration or loss Stratum granulosum • Granular layer • Responsible for keratin formation Stratum spinosum • Spiny layer • Helps with keratin formation • Contains a rich supply of ribonucleic acid Stratum basale (basal layer) • Innermost layer • Produces new superficial cells
Dermis • Also called the *corium* • Contains and supports blood vessels, lymphatic vessels, nerves, and the epidermal appendages • Composed primarily of matrix, which contains collagen (gives strength), elastin (provides elasticity), and reticular fibers (bind collagen and elastin fibers together) • Consists of two sublayers	 Papillary dermis • Contains fingerlike projections (papillae) that connect the dermis to the epidermis • Contains characteristic ridges Reticular dermis • Covers a layer of subcutaneous tissue, insulating the body to conserve heat • Provides energy • Serves as a mechanical shock absorber

Cross-section of the skin

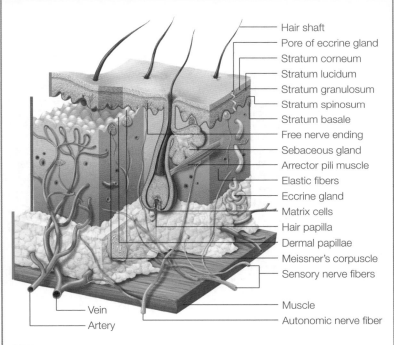

- Hair shaft
- Pore of eccrine gland
- Stratum corneum
- Stratum lucidum
- Stratum granulosum
- Stratum spinosum
- Stratum basale
- Free nerve ending
- Sebaceous gland
- Arrector pili muscle
- Elastic fibers
- Eccrine gland
- Matrix cells
- Hair papilla
- Dermal papillae
- Meissner's corpuscle
- Sensory nerve fibers
- Muscle
- Autonomic nerve fiber
- Vein
- Artery

Key

- Epidermis
- Dermis
- Subcutaneous tissue

Skin functions

- Performs many vital functions
- Has a role in protection, sensory perception, excretion, and regulation of body temperature

Protection	Sensory perception	Excretion	Body temperature
• Maintains the integrity of the body surface (through skin migration and shedding) • Repairs surface wounds (by intensifying normal cell replacement) • Protects the body against noxious chemicals and invasion from bacteria and microorganisms • Contains Langerhans' cells (specialized cells in the skin's top layer) that enhance the body's immune response • Contains melanocytes (which produce the brown pigment melanin) that help filter ultraviolet light	• Contains sensory nerve fibers that supply specific areas of the skin (dermatomes) • Allows for perception of temperature, touch, pressure, pain, and itching • Contains autonomic nerve fibers that carry impulses to smooth muscle in the walls of the skin's blood vessels, to the muscles around the hair roots, and to the sweat glands	• Excretes sweat, which contains water, electrolytes, urea, and lactic acid • Prevents dehydration by regulating the content and volume of sweat • Prevents unwanted fluids in the environment from entering the body	• Contains nerves, blood vessels, and eccrine glands within the skin's deeper layer to control body temperature • Causes blood vessels to constrict (reducing blood flow and conserving heat) when exposed to cold or internal body temperature falls • Causes small arteries within the skin to dilate (increasing the blood flow and reducing body heat) when skin becomes too hot or internal body temperature rises

How melanocytes protect skin from ultraviolet light

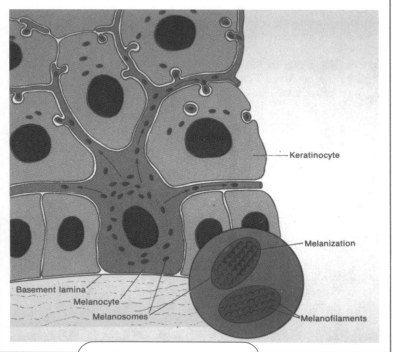

Keratinocyte

Melanization

Basement lamina
Melanocyte
Melanosomes

Melanofilaments

As you recall, melanocytes produce a brown pigment, melanin, which helps filter out ultraviolet light. They do this by transferring the melanin granules to keratinocytes in the epidermal layer. Pretty cool, huh?

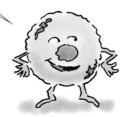

Hair

- Consists of long, slender shafts composed of keratin
- Contains a bulb or root at the expanded lower end of each hair
- Indented by a *hair papilla* (a cluster of connective tissue and blood vessels) on its undersurface
- Lies within an epithelium-lined sheath called a *hair follicle*
- Extending through the dermis to attach to the base of the follicle are *arrector pili* (a bundle of smooth-muscle fibers)
- When these muscles contract, hair stands on end
- Hair follicles have a rich blood and nerve supply

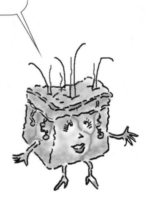

A close look at hair

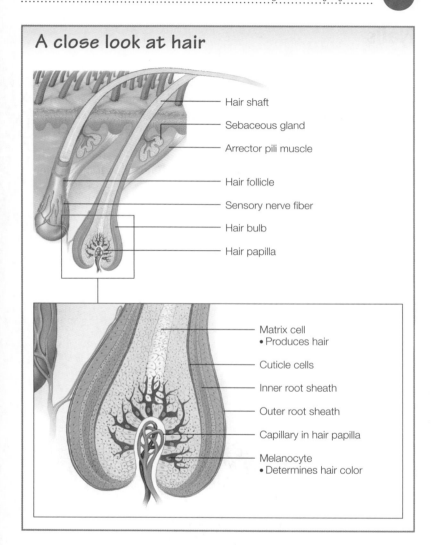

- Hair shaft
- Sebaceous gland
- Arrector pili muscle
- Hair follicle
- Sensory nerve fiber
- Hair bulb
- Hair papilla

- Matrix cell
  • Produces hair
- Cuticle cells
- Inner root sheath
- Outer root sheath
- Capillary in hair papilla
- Melanocyte
  • Determines hair color

Nails

- Situated over the distal surface of the end of each finger and toe
- Composed of a specialized type of keratin
- Covering the nail bed is a *nail plate* (formed by the nail matrix, which extends proximally for about ¼″ [0.5 cm] beneath the nail fold)
- Surrounding three sides of the nail plate are nail folds, or *cuticles*
- The distal portion of the matrix shows through the nail as a pale crescent-moon–shaped area, called the *lunula*
- The translucent nail plate distal to the lunula exposes the nail bed
- The vascular bed imparts the characteristic pink appearance under the nails

It's hard to believe that nails are just a specialized type of keratin, the same kind of cells that make up skin and hair.

A close look at nails

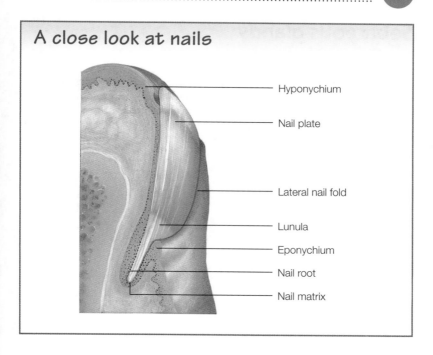

Hyponychium

Nail plate

Lateral nail fold

Lunula

Eponychium

Nail root

Nail matrix

Sebaceous glands

- Are part of the hair follicle and occur on all parts of the skin except the palms and soles
- Are most prominent on the scalp, face, upper torso, and genitalia
- Produce *sebum*, a mixture of keratin, fat, and cellulose debris
  - Forms a moist, oily, acidic film (when combined with sweat) that's mildly antibacterial and antifungal and that protects the skin surface
  - Exits through the hair follicle opening to reach the skin surface

A close look at sebaceous glands

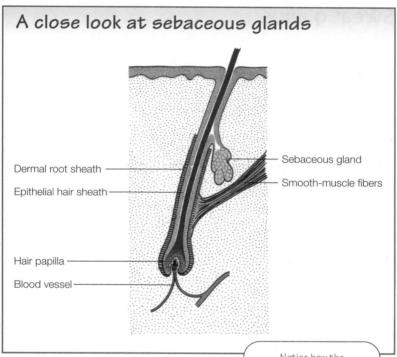

Dermal root sheath

Epithelial hair sheath

Hair papilla

Blood vessel

Sebaceous gland

Smooth-muscle fibers

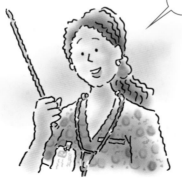

Notice how the sebaceous gland lies proximal to the hair follicle, through which sebum exits to reach the skin surface.

Sweat glands

- Consist of two types: eccrine glands and apocrine glands
- Purpose and function of two types varies

Eccrine glands

- Are widely distributed throughout the body
- Produce an odorless, watery fluid with a sodium concentration equal to that of plasma
- Opens onto the skin surface via a duct extending from the coiled secretory portion through the dermis and epidermis
- Function varies according to location
  - Eccrine glands in the palms and soles secrete fluid mainly in response to emotional stress
  - The remaining three million eccrine glands respond primarily to thermal stress, effectively regulating temperature
- Found everywhere except the lips and glans penis

Apocrine glands

- Located chiefly in the axillary (underarm) and anogenital (groin) areas
- Have a coiled secretory portion that lies deeper in the dermis than that of the eccrine glands
- Connected to the upper portion of the hair follicle by a duct
- Begin to function at puberty
- Have no known biological function
- Produce body odor as bacteria decompose the fluids secreted by these glands

A closer look at sweat glands

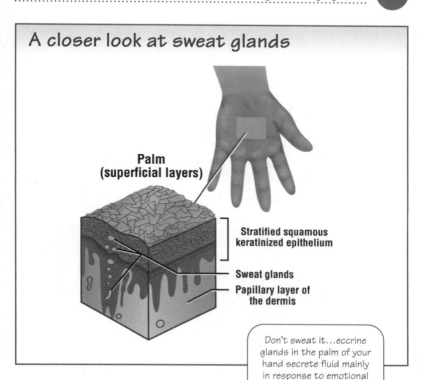

**Palm
(superficial layers)**

Stratified squamous
keratinized epithelium

Sweat glands

Papillary layer of
the dermis

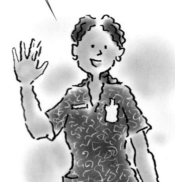

Don't sweat it...eccrine
glands in the palm of your
hand secrete fluid mainly
in response to emotional
stress.

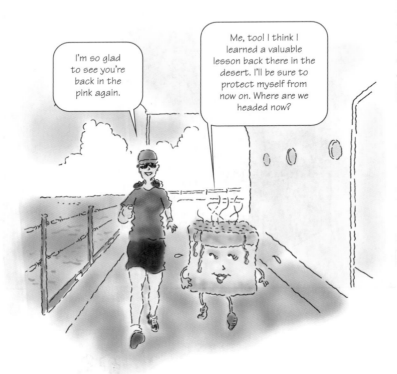

5

Musculoskeletal system

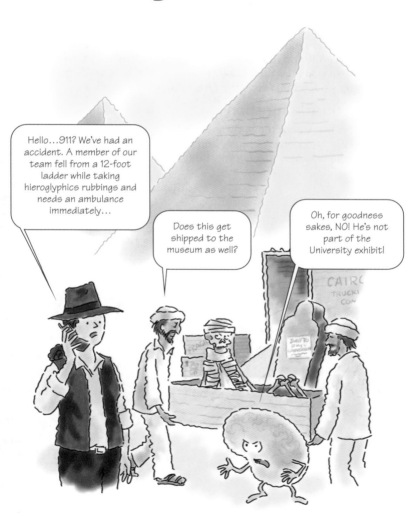

Musculoskeletal system basics

- Consists of muscles, tendons, ligaments, bones, cartilage, joints, and bursae
- Gives the human body its shape and ability to move

Muscles

- Classified by the tissue they contain:
    - *Cardiac* (heart) muscle: consists of a specialized type of striated tissue
    - *Smooth* (involuntary) muscle: contains smooth-muscle tissue
    - *Skeletal* (voluntary and reflex) muscle: consists of striated tissue
- The human body has about 600 skeletal muscles. (This chapter discusses only skeletal muscle—the type attached to bone.)

Skeletal muscle function

- Moves body parts or the body as a whole
- Responsible for both voluntary and reflex movements
- Maintains posture and generates body heat

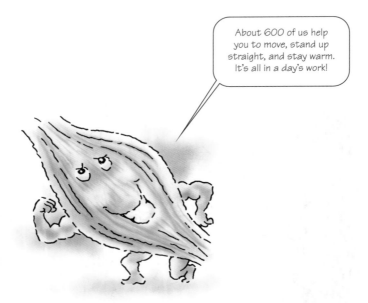

(Text continues on page 74.)

Major skeletal muscles (anterior view)

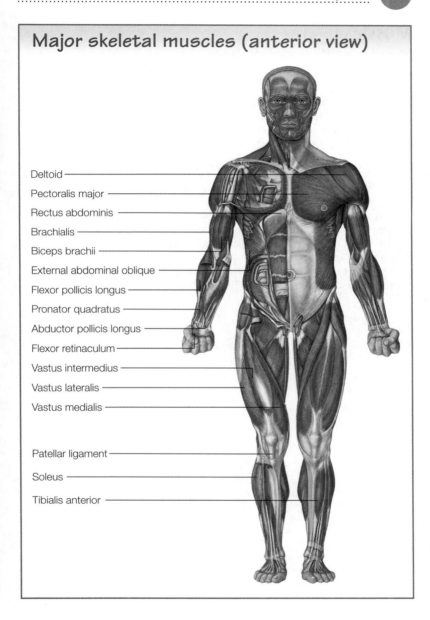

Deltoid

Pectoralis major

Rectus abdominis

Brachialis

Biceps brachii

External abdominal oblique

Flexor pollicis longus

Pronator quadratus

Abductor pollicis longus

Flexor retinaculum

Vastus intermedius

Vastus lateralis

Vastus medialis

Patellar ligament

Soleus

Tibialis anterior

Muscles *(continued)*

Muscles of the axial skeleton

- Essential for respiration, speech, facial expression, posture, and chewing
- Muscles of axial skeleton include:
  - muscles of the face, tongue, and neck
  - muscles of mastication
  - muscles of the vertebral column situated along the spine

Muscles of the appendicular skeleton

- These include:
  - muscles of the shoulder
  - muscles of the abdominopelvic cavity
  - muscles of the upper and lower extremities
- Muscles of the upper extremities are classified according to the bones they move
- Those that move the arm are further categorized into those with an origin on the axial skeleton and those with an origin on the scapula

(Text continues on page 76.)

Major skeletal muscles (posterior view)

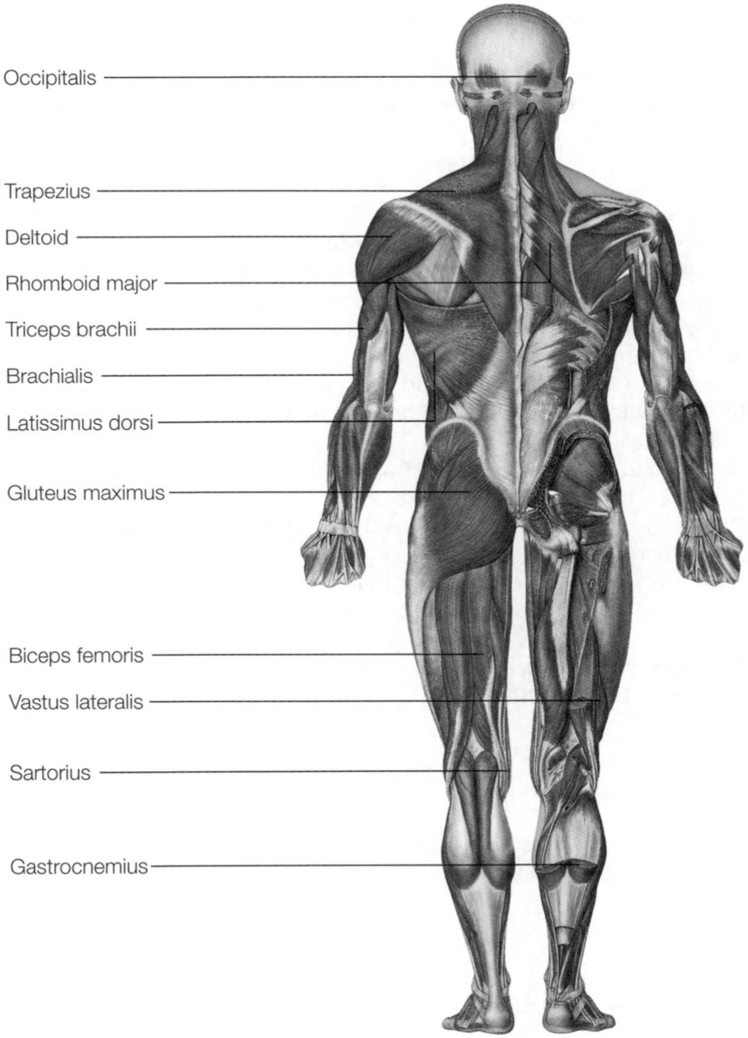

Occipitalis

Trapezius

Deltoid

Rhomboid major

Triceps brachii

Brachialis

Latissimus dorsi

Gluteus maximus

Biceps femoris

Vastus lateralis

Sartorius

Gastrocnemius

Muscles *(continued)*

Skeletal muscle structure

- Composed of large, long cells called *muscle fibers*
- Each fiber has many nuclei and a series of increasingly smaller internal fibrous structures
- Structures of a muscle fiber (working from the cell's exterior to its interior) are:
  - *endomysium*—the connective tissue layer surrounding an individual skeletal muscle fiber
  - *sarcolemma*—the plasma membrane of the cell that lies beneath the endomysium and just above the cell's nucleus
  - *sarcoplasm*—the muscle cell's cytoplasm, which is contained within the sarcolemma
  - *myofibrils*—tiny, threadlike structures that run the fiber's length and make up the bulk of the fiber
  - *myosin* (thick filaments) and *actin* (thin filaments)—still finer fibers within the myofibrils; there are about 1,500 myosin and about 3,000 actin
- Myosin and actin are contained within compartments called *sarcomeres*
- During muscle contraction, myosin and actin slide over each other, reducing sarcomere length
- A fibrous sheath of connective tissue, called the *perimysium*, binds muscle fibers into a bundle, or *fascicle*
- A stronger sheath, the *epimysium*, binds all of the fascicles together to form the entire muscle
- Extending beyond the muscle, the epimysium becomes a tendon

(Text continues on page 78.)

Muscle structure

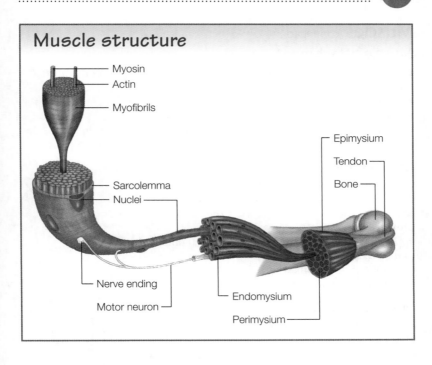

- Myosin
- Actin
- Myofibrils
- Sarcolemma
- Nuclei
- Nerve ending
- Motor neuron
- Endomysium
- Perimysium
- Epimysium
- Tendon
- Bone

Muscles *(continued)*
Muscle attachment

● Most skeletal muscles are attached to bones (either directly or indirectly)
● Direct attachment: the epimysium of the muscle fuses to the *periosteum*, the fibrous membrane covering the bone
● Indirect attachment (most common): the epimysium extends past the muscle as a tendon, or *aponeurosis*, and attaches to the bone

Contraction

● During contraction, one of the bones to which the muscle is attached stays relatively stationary while the other is pulled in toward the stationary one
● *Origin:* the point where the muscle attaches to the stationary or less movable bone
● *Insertion:* the point where the muscle attaches to the more movable bone

Muscle growth

● Muscle develops when existing muscle fibers hypertrophy
● Muscle strength and size differ among individuals because of such factors as exercise, nutrition, gender, age, and genetic constitution

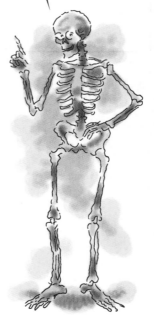

When a muscle contracts, it pulls one bone toward another bone that's relatively stationary.

(Text continues on page 80.)

Understanding indirect muscle attachment

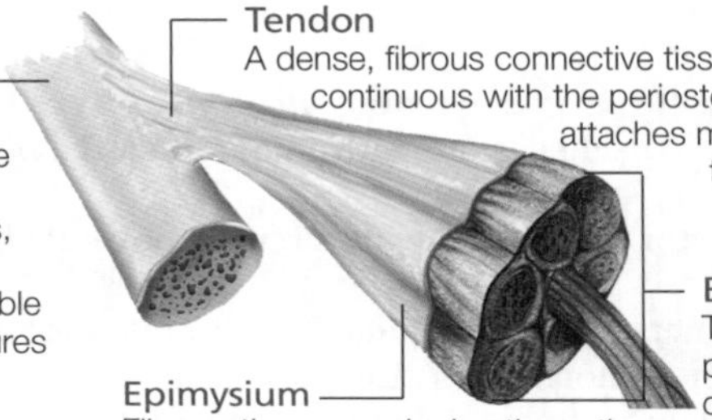

Tendon
A dense, fibrous connective tissue that's continuous with the periosteum and attaches muscle to the bone

Periosteum
A tough, fibrous connective tissue that covers the surface of bones, rich in sensory nerves, responsible for healing fractures

Belly
Thick contractile portion (or body) of the muscle

Epimysium
Fibrous tissue enveloping the entire muscle and continuous with the tendon

Muscles *(continued)*

Muscle movements

- Skeletal muscle permits several types of movement
- A muscle's functional name comes from the type of movement it permits
  - A flexor muscle permits bending *(flexion)*
  - An adductor muscle permits movement toward a body axis *(adduction)*
  - A circumductor muscle allows a circular movement *(circumduction)*
- Diarthrodial joints allow 13 angular and circular movements:
  - The shoulder demonstrates circumduction
  - The elbow demonstrates flexion and extension
  - The hip demonstrates internal and external rotation
  - The arm demonstrates abduction and adduction
  - The hand demonstrates supination and pronation
  - The jaw demonstrates retraction and protraction
  - The foot demonstrates eversion and inversion.

Basic body movements

Retraction and protraction
Moving backward and forward

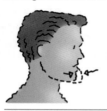

Flexion
Bending, decreasing the joint angle

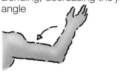

Extension
Straightening, increasing the joint angle

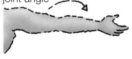

Circumduction
Moving in a circular motion

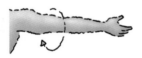

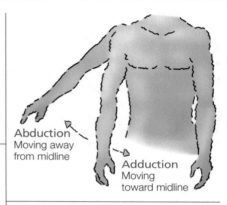

Abduction
Moving away from midline

Adduction
Moving toward midline

Internal rotation
Turning toward midline

External rotation
Turning away from midline

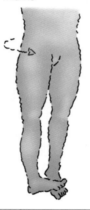

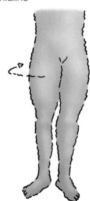

Pronation
Turning downward

Supination
Turning upward

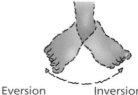

Eversion
Turning outward

Inversion
Turning inward

Tendons, ligaments, and bones

- *Tendons*: bands of fibrous connective tissue that attach muscles to the periosteum (the fibrous covering of bone)
- Tendons enable bones to move when skeletal muscles contract
- *Ligaments*: dense, strong, flexible bands of fibrous connective tissue that bind bones to other bones
- *Bones*: form the human skeleton (which contains 206 bones)
  - The *axial skeleton* (which lies along the central line, or axis, of the body) is composed of 80 bones
  - The bones of the axial skeleton include facial and cranial bones, vertebrae, hyoid bone, ribs, and sternum
  - The *appendicular skeleton* (relating to the limbs, or appendages, of the body) is composed of 126 bones
  - Bones of the appendicular skeleton include the clavicle, pelvic bones, scapula, humerus, radius, ulna, carpals, metacarpals, phalanges, femur, patella, fibula, tibia, tarsals, metatarsals, and phalanges

(Text continues on page 84.)

Major bones (anterior view)

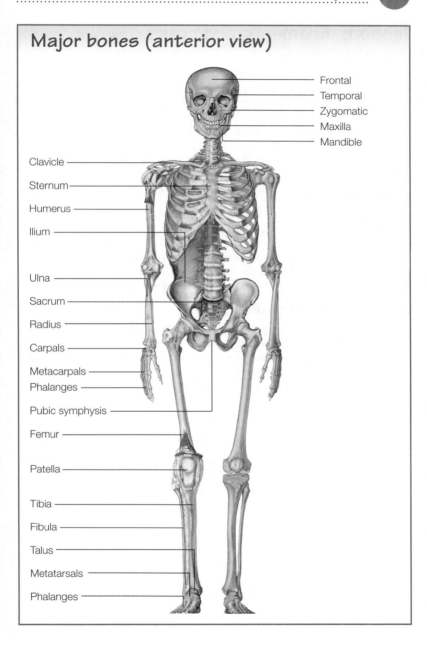

Frontal
Temporal
Zygomatic
Maxilla
Mandible

Clavicle
Sternum
Humerus
Ilium

Ulna
Sacrum
Radius
Carpals
Metacarpals
Phalanges
Pubic symphysis
Femur

Patella

Tibia
Fibula
Talus
Metatarsals
Phalanges

Tendons, ligaments, and bones *(continued)*

Bone classification

- Bones are typically classified by shape
- Bone classifications include:
  - long (such as the humerus, radius, femur, and tibia)
  - short (such as the carpals and tarsals)
  - flat (such as the scapula, ribs, and skull)
  - irregular (such as the vertebrae and mandible)
  - sesamoid, which is a small bone developed in a tendon (such as the patella)

Bone functions

- Bones protect internal tissues and organs
- They stabilize and support the body
- They provide a surface for muscle, ligament, and tendon attachment
- Bones move through "lever" action when contracted
- They produce red blood cells in the bone marrow (hematopoiesis)
- Bones store mineral salts (such as 99% of the body's calcium)

Blood supply to the bones

- *Haversian canals* (minute channels that lie parallel to the axis of the bone) are passages for arterioles
- *Volkmann's canals* contain vessels that connect one haversian canal to another and to the outer bone
- *Vessels* exist in the bone ends and within the marrow

(Text continues on page 86.)

Major bones (posterior view)

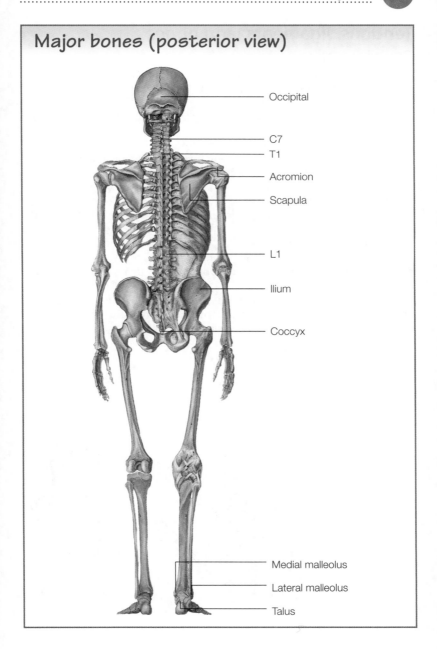

Occipital

C7

T1

Acromion

Scapula

L1

Ilium

Coccyx

Medial malleolus

Lateral malleolus

Talus

Tendons, ligaments, and bones *(continued)*

Bone formation

- At 3 months in utero, the fetal skeleton is composed of cartilage
- By about 6 months, fetal cartilage has been transformed into bony skeleton
- After birth, some bones (most notably the carpals and tarsals) *ossify* (harden)
  - The change results from *endochondral ossification*
  - In this process, *osteoblasts* (bone-forming cells) produce *osteoid* (a collagenous material that ossifies)

Bone remodeling

- *Remodeling*: the continuous process whereby bone is created and destroyed
- *Osteoblasts* deposit new bone
- *Osteoclasts* increase long-bone diameter
- Osteoclasts promote longitudinal bone growth by reabsorbing previously deposited bone
- Longitudinal growth continues until the *epiphyseal plates* (cartilage that separate the *diaphysis*, or shaft of a bone, from the *epiphysis*, or end of a bone) ossify during late adolescence

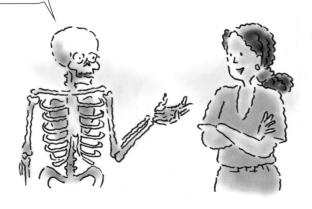

My mother wanted me to become an interior decorator...she said I had a real knack for remodeling.

Stages of bone growth and remodeling

1.
Creation of an ossification center

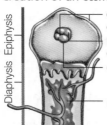

Epiphysis | Diaphysis

- Growing hyaline cartilage
- Enlarged cartilage cells
- Cavities
- Medullary cavity

2.
Osteoblasts form bone

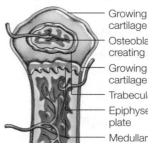

- Growing cartilage
- Osteoblasts creating bone
- Growing cartilage
- Trabeculae
- Epiphyseal plate
- Medullary cavity

3.
Bone length grows

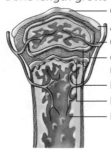

- Growing cartilage
- Articular cartilage
- Ossifying cartilage
- Compact bone replacing cartilage
- Epiphyseal plate
- New trabeculae
- Medullary cavity

4.
Remodeling

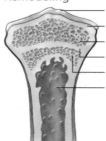

- Articular cartilage
- Compact bone
- Cancellous bone
- Epiphyseal line
- Cancellous bone
- Medullary cavity

Cartilage

- A dense connective tissue consisting of fibers embedded in a strong, gel-like substance
- Supports and shapes various structures
- Cushions and absorbs shock, preventing direct transmission to the bone
- Has no blood supply or innervation
- Consists of three types: *hyaline, fibrous,* and *elastic*

Hyaline cartilage

- The most common type
- Covers the articular bone surfaces (where one or more bones meet at a joint)
- Connects the ribs to the sternum and appears in the trachea, bronchi, and nasal septum

Fibrous cartilage

- Forms the symphysis pubis and the intervertebral disks
- Composed of small quantities of matrix and abundant fibrous elements
- Strong and rigid

Elastic cartilage

- The most pliable cartilage
- Located in the auditory canal, external ear, and epiglottis
- Elastic and resilient

A close look at cartilage

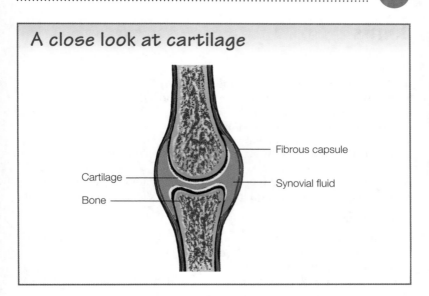

Fibrous capsule

Cartilage

Synovial fluid

Bone

Joints

- *Joints* (articulations): points of contact between two bones that hold the bones together
- May also allow flexibility and movement
- May be classified by function (extent of movement):
  - *synarthrosis* (immovable)
  - *amphiarthrosis* (slightly movable)
  - *diarthrosis* (freely movable)
- May also be classified by structure (what they're made of): *fibrous, cartilaginous,* or *synovial*
- Based on structure and type of movement, synovial joints may be classified as gliding, hinge, pivot, condylar, saddle, and ball-and-socket

Bursae

- Small synovial fluid sacs located at friction points around joints between tendons, ligaments, and bones
- Act as cushions to decrease stress on adjacent structures
- Examples: the subacromial bursa (located in the shoulder) and the prepatellar bursa (located in the knee)

> Some common examples of synovial joints are hinge joints (like knees and elbows), gliding joints (like ankles, wrists, and the spine), pivot joints (like the neck), and ball-and-socket joints (like the shoulders and me).

Common joints

Joint type		Description
Ball-and-socket joint		• Located in the shoulders and hips • Allow flexion, extension, adduction, and abduction • Rotate in their sockets • Assessed by their degrees of internal and external rotation
Hinge joint		• Include the knee and the elbow • Move in flexion and extension
Pivot joint		• Rounded portion of one bone in a pivot joint fits into a groove in another bone • Allow only uniaxial rotation of the first bone around the second • Includes the head of the radius, which rotates within a groove of the ulna
Condylar joint		• An oval surface of one bone fits into a concavity in another bone • Allow flexion, extension, abduction, adduction, and circumduction • Includes the radiocarpal and metacarpophalangeal joints of the hand
Saddle joint		• Resemble condylar joints but allow greater freedom of movement • Only saddle joints are the carpometacarpal joints of the thumb

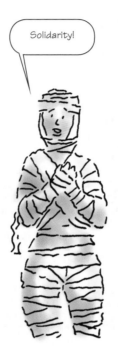

6

Neurosensory system

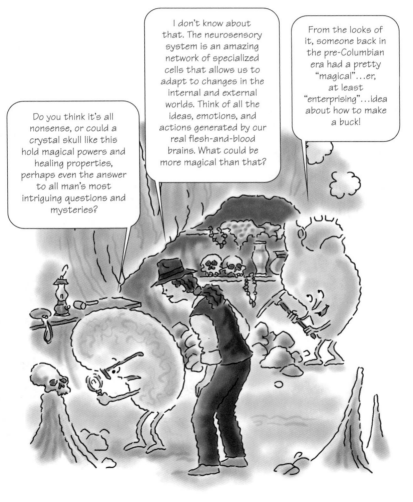

Neurosensory system basics

- Coordinates all body functions
- Enables a person to adapt to changes in internal and external environments
- Has two main types of cells: *neurons* (conducting cells) and *neuroglia* (supportive cells)

Neuron

- The basic unit of the nervous system
- Receives and transmits electrochemical nerve impulses
- Has *axons* and *dendrites* extending from the central cell body; typically has one axon and many dendrites

Axons

- Conduct nerve impulses away from cell bodies
- Typically have terminal branches and are wrapped in a myelin sheath, which is produced by *Schwann cells* (phagocytic cells separated by gaps called nodes of Ranvier)

Dendrites

- Conduct impulses toward the cell body
- Receive impulses from other cells

Neuroglia

- Also called *glial cells*
- Form about 40% of brain's bulk

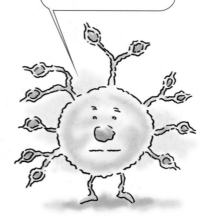

My dendrites act like receivers, pulling impulses toward my cell body, while my axon conducts the impulses away from me to the next cell in line.

(Text continues on page 96.)

Parts of a neuron

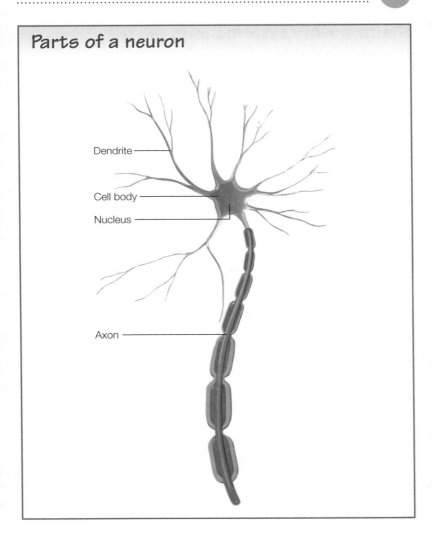

Dendrite

Cell body

Nucleus

Axon

Neurosensory system basics *(continued)*
Neurotransmission
- Defined as the conduction of electrochemical impulses throughout the nervous system
- Performed by neurons, which may be provoked by:
  - mechanical stimuli (such as touch and pressure)
  - thermal stimuli (such as heat and cold)
  - chemical stimuli (such as external chemicals or a chemical released by the body, such as histamine)

The reflex arc
- A neural relay cycle for quick motor response to a harmful sensory stimulus
- Requires a sensory (*afferent*) neuron and a motor (*efferent*) neuron
- Triggered by a stimulus, which transmits a sensory impulse along the dorsal root to the spinal cord
- Causes two simultaneous synaptic transmissions
  - One synapse continues the impulse along a sensory neuron to the brain
  - The other synapse immediately relays the impulse to an interneuron, which transmits it to a motor neuron

How neurotransmission occurs

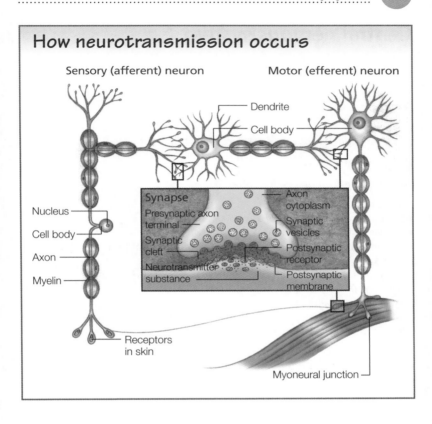

Sensory (afferent) neuron

Motor (efferent) neuron

Dendrite

Cell body

Nucleus

Cell body

Axon

Myelin

Synapse

Presynaptic axon terminal

Synaptic cleft

Neurotransmitter substance

Axon cytoplasm

Synaptic vesicles

Postsynaptic receptor

Postsynaptic membrane

Receptors in skin

Myoneural junction

Central nervous system

- Includes the brain and the spinal cord
- Encased by the bones of the skull and the vertebral column
- Protected by cerebral spinal fluid and the meninges

Brain

- Consists of the cerebrum, cerebellum, brain stem, diencephalon (thalamus and hypothalamus), limbic system, and reticular activating system
- Works with the spinal cord to collect and interpret voluntary and involuntary motor and sensory stimuli

Cerebrum

- Also known as the *cerebral cortex*
- Controls the ability to think and reason
- Enclosed by three meninges (dura mater, arachnoid mater, and pia mater)
- Contains the diencephalon, which consists of the *thalamus* and *hypothalamus*
  - Thalamus: acts as the relay station for sensory impulses
  - Hypothalamus: controls regulatory functions, including body temperature, pituitary hormone production, and water balance

Brain stem

- Contains the midbrain, pons, and medulla oblongata
- Regulates autonomic body functions, such as heart rate, breathing, and swallowing
- Contains cranial nerves III through XII

Cerebellum

- Contains major motor and sensory pathways
- Helps maintain equilibrium
- Controls muscle coordination

(Text continues on page 100.)

The brain

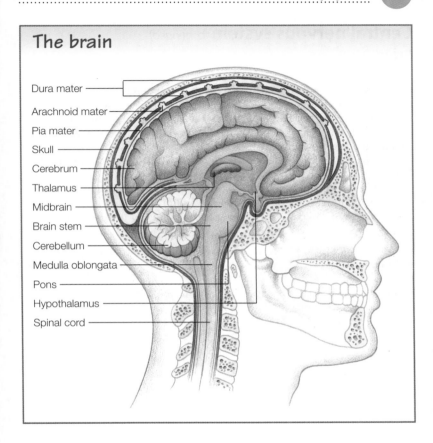

Dura mater

Arachnoid mater

Pia mater

Skull

Cerebrum

Thalamus

Midbrain

Brain stem

Cerebellum

Medulla oblongata

Pons

Hypothalamus

Spinal cord

Central nervous system *(continued)*

Brain *(continued)*

Cerebral lobes

- Consist of four divisions of each cerebral hemisphere
- Based on anatomic landmarks and functional differences
  - *Parietal lobe*: interprets and integrates sensation (including touch, pain, and temperature); contributes to understanding of speech and language and thought expression
  - *Occipital lobe*: contributes to visual recognition and focus of the eye
  - *Frontal lobe*: influences motor control of voluntary muscles, personality, concentration, organization, and problem-solving
  - *Temporal lobe*: controls hearing and memory of hearing and vision

Limbic system

- Consists of a primitive brain area deep within the temporal lobe
- Initiates basic drives (such as hunger, aggression, and emotional and sexual arousal)
- Screens all sensory messages traveling to the cerebral cortex

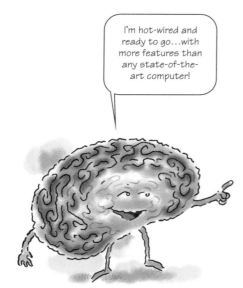

I'm hot-wired and ready to go…with more features than any state-of-the-art computer!

(Text continues on page 102.)

Cerebral lobes

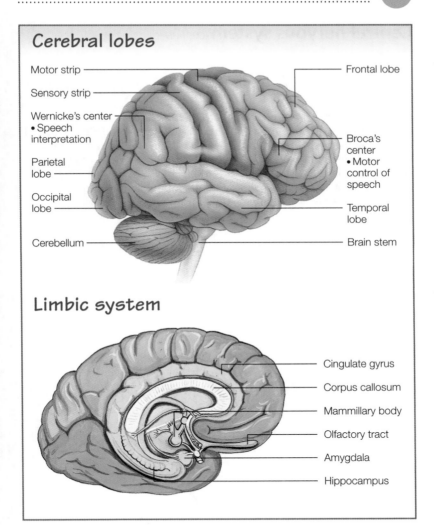

Motor strip
Sensory strip
Wernicke's center
• Speech interpretation
Parietal lobe
Occipital lobe
Cerebellum

Frontal lobe
Broca's center
• Motor control of speech
Temporal lobe
Brain stem

Limbic system

Cingulate gyrus
Corpus callosum
Mammillary body
Olfactory tract
Amygdala
Hippocampus

Central nervous system *(continued)*

Brain *(continued)*

Oxygenating the brain

- Two *vertebral arteries* (branches of the subclavians) converge to become the basilar artery
- The *basilar artery* supplies blood to the posterior brain
- The common carotids branch into the two internal carotids, which divide further to supply blood to the anterior brain and the middle brain
- These arteries interconnect through the *circle of Willis*, an anastomosis at the base of the brain
- The circle of Willis ensures that blood continually circulates to the brain despite interruption of any of the brain's major vessels

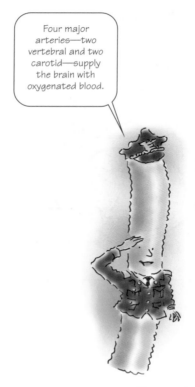

Four major arteries—two vertebral and two carotid—supply the brain with oxygenated blood.

(Text continues on page 104.)

Arteries of the brain

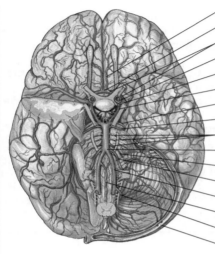

Medial orbitofrontal artery
Anterior communicating artery
Anterior cerebral artery
Internal carotid artery
Middle cerebral artery
Posterior communicating artery
Posterior cerebral artery
Superior cerebellar artery
Pontine arteries
Basilar artery
Internal acoustic artery
Anterior inferior cerebellar artery
Vertebral artery
Anterior spinal artery
Posterior spinal artery
Transverse sinus

Circle of Willis

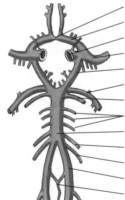

Anterior communicating artery
Anterior cerebral artery
Internal carotid artery
Middle cerebral artery
Posterior communicating artery
Posterior cerebral artery
Superior cerebellar artery
Pontine arteries
Basilar artery
Internal acoustic artery
Anterior inferior cerebellar artery
Vertebral artery
Anterior spinal artery
Posterior spinal artery

Central nervous system *(continued)*

The spinal cord

- A cylindrical structure in the vertebral canal
- Extends from the foramen magnum at the base of the skull to the upper lumbar region of the vertebral column
- Gives rise to the spinal nerves
- Contains an H-shaped mass of gray matter that is divided into *horns*
  - Horns consist mainly of neuron cell bodies
  - Cell bodies in the two *dorsal* (posterior) horns primarily relay sensations
  - Those in the two *ventral* (anterior) horns play a part in voluntary and reflex motor activity
- Surrounded by white matter
  - This white matter consists of myelinated nerve fibers grouped in vertical columns, or *tracts*
  - All axons that compose one tract serve one general function (such as touch, movement, pain, and pressure)

A look inside the spinal cord

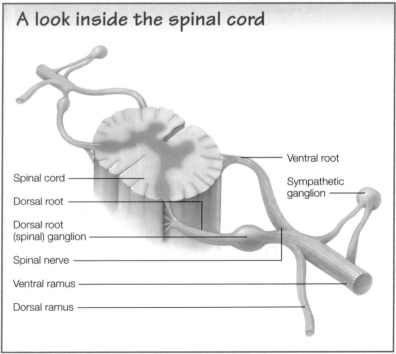

(Text continues on page 106.)

Spinal cord

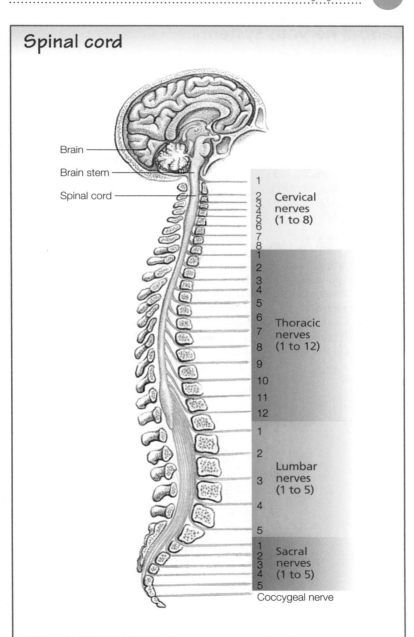

Brain

Brain stem

Spinal cord

1
2
3
4
5
6
7
8
Cervical nerves (1 to 8)

1
2
3
4
5
6
7
8
9
10
11
12
Thoracic nerves (1 to 12)

1
2
3
4
5
Lumbar nerves (1 to 5)

1
2
3
4
5
Sacral nerves (1 to 5)

Coccygeal nerve

Central nervous system *(continued)*
Neural pathways
Sensory pathways
● Conduct sensory impulses via the *afferent* (ascending) neural pathways to the sensory cortex in the parietal lobe
● Impulses travel up the cord in the dorsal column to the medulla, then cross to the opposite side and into the thalamus
● The thalamus then relays all incoming sensory impulses (except olfactory impulses) to the sensory cortex for interpretation
● Pain and temperature sensations enter through the dorsal horn; touch, pressure, vibration, and pain sensations enter via relay stations called *ganglia* (knotlike masses of nerve cell bodies on the dorsal roots of spinal nerves)

Motor pathways
● Conduct motor impulses from the brain to the muscles via the *efferent* (descending) neural pathways
● Motor impulses originate in the motor cortex of the frontal lobe and reach the lower motor neurons of the peripheral nervous system via upper motor neurons
● Upper motor neurons originate in the brain and form two major systems: the pyramidal system (fine motor movements) and the extrapyramidal system (gross motor movements)

(Text continues on page 108.)

Major neural pathways

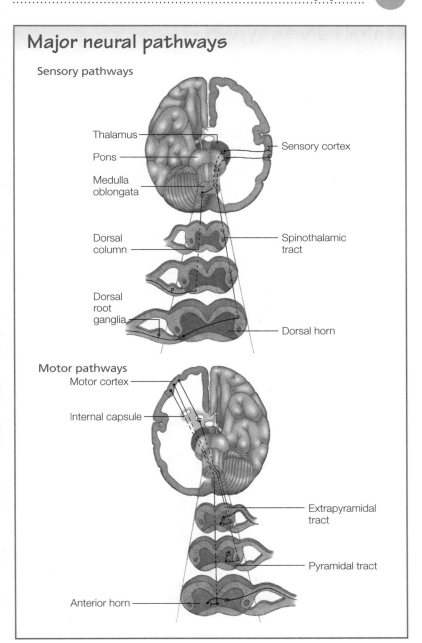

Sensory pathways

Thalamus

Pons

Medulla oblongata

Sensory cortex

Dorsal column

Spinothalamic tract

Dorsal root ganglia

Dorsal horn

Motor pathways

Motor cortex

Internal capsule

Extrapyramidal tract

Pyramidal tract

Anterior horn

Central nervous system *(continued)*
Neural pathways *(continued)*

Reflex responses
- Occur automatically, without any brain involvement
- Purpose is to protect the body
- *Superficial reflexes* – consist of withdrawal reflexes elicited by noxious or tactile stimulation of the skin or mucous membranes
- *Primitive reflexes* – considered abnormal in adults, but normal in infants
- *Deep tendon reflexes* – involve involuntary contractions of a muscle after brief stretching caused by tendon percussion; include:
  - *Biceps reflex*: contracts the biceps muscle and forces flexion of the forearm
  - *Triceps reflex*: contracts the triceps muscle and forces extension of the forearm
  - *Brachioradialis reflex*: causes supination of the hand and flexion of the forearm at the elbow
  - *Patellar reflex*: forces contraction of the quadriceps muscle in the thigh with extension of the leg
  - *Achilles reflex*: forces plantar flexion of the foot at the ankle

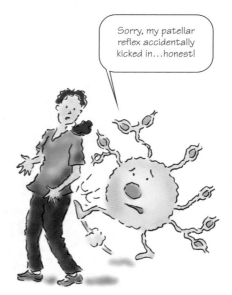

Sorry, my patellar reflex accidentally kicked in...honest!

(Text continues on page 110.)

Eliciting deep tendon reflexes

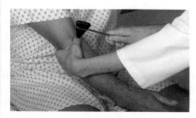

Biceps reflex
Position the patient's arm so his elbow is flexed at a 45-degree angle and his arm is relaxed. Place your thumb or index finger over the biceps tendon. Strike your finger with the pointed end of the reflex hammer.

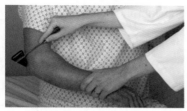

Triceps reflex
Ask the patient to adduct his arm and place his forearm across his chest. Strike the triceps tendon about 2″ (5 cm) above the olecranon process on the extensor surface of the upper arm.

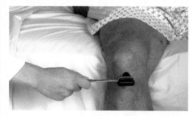

Patellar reflex
Ask the patient to sit with his legs dangling freely. If he can't sit up, flex his knee at a 45-degree angle and place your nondominant hand behind it for support. Strike the patellar tendon just below the patella.

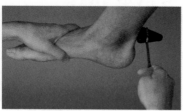

Achilles reflex
Ask the patient to flex his foot. Strike the Achilles tendon.

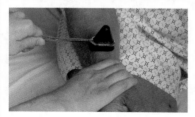

Brachioradialis reflex
Ask the patient to rest the ulnar surface of his hand on his abdomen or lap with the elbow partially flexed. Strike the radius.

Central nervous system *(continued)*

Protective structures

● *Meninges*: membranous coverings that help protect the brain and spinal cord

● *Dura mater*: tough, fibrous, leatherlike tissue composed of the *endosteal dura* (forms the periosteum of the skull and is continuous with the lining of the vertebral canal) and the *meningeal dura* (a thick membrane that covers the brain, providing support and protection)

● *Subdural space*: lies between the dura mater and the arachnoid membrane

● *Arachnoid membrane*: thin, fibrous membrane that hugs the brain and spinal cord

● *Subarachnoid space*: lies between the arachnoid membrane and the pia mater

● *Pia mater*: continuous, delicate layer of connective tissue that covers and contours the spinal tissue and brain

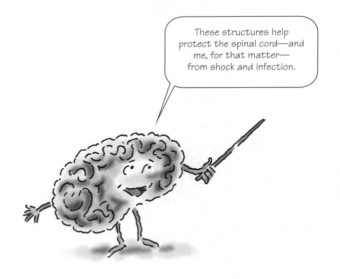

These structures help protect the spinal cord—and me, for that matter—from shock and infection.

The meninges

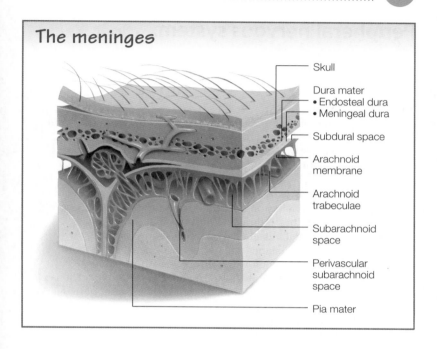

Skull

Dura mater
• Endosteal dura
• Meningeal dura

Subdural space

Arachnoid membrane

Arachnoid trabeculae

Subarachnoid space

Perivascular subarachnoid space

Pia mater

Peripheral nervous system

- Extends outside the CNS
- Consists of the cranial nerves (CN), spinal nerves, and autonomic nervous system (ANS)

Cranial nerves

- Serve as primary motor and sensory pathways between the brain, head, and neck
- Consist of 12 pairs of nerves
  - *Olfactory*: smell
  - *Optic*: vision
  - *Oculomotor, trochlear,* and *abducens*: extraocular eye movements
  - *Trigeminal*: transmission of stimuli from face and head, corneal reflex, chewing, biting, lateral jaw movements
  - *Facial*: taste, facial muscle movements (expression)
  - *Acoustic*: hearing, balance
  - *Glossopharyngeal*: swallowing, throat sensations, taste
  - *Vagus*: movement of palate, swallowing, gag, activity and sensations of the thoracic and abdominal viscera (heart rate, peristalsis), sensations of throat and larynx
  - *Spinal accessory*: shoulder movement, head rotation
  - *Hypoglossal*: tongue movement

(Text continues on page 114.)

Exit points for the cranial nerves

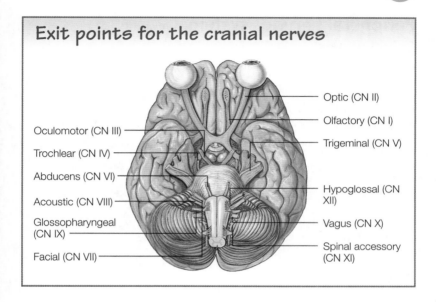

Optic (CN II)

Olfactory (CN I)

Oculomotor (CN III)

Trigeminal (CN V)

Trochlear (CN IV)

Abducens (CN VI)

Hypoglossal (CN XII)

Acoustic (CN VIII)

Glossopharyngeal (CN IX)

Vagus (CN X)

Facial (CN VII)

Spinal accessory (CN XI)

Peripheral nervous system *(continued)*

Spinal nerves

● Arise from the spinal cord; at the cord's inferior end, nerve roots cluster in the *cauda equina*

● Composed of 31 pairs, each named for the vertebra immediately below the nerve's exit point from the spinal cord

● Designated as C1 through S5 and the coccygeal nerve (from top to bottom)

● Consists of afferent (sensory) and efferent (motor) neurons, which carry messages to and from particular body regions, called *dermatomes*

● Mediate the deep tendon reflexes, superficial reflexes, and primitive reflexes

● Many nerves join together to form networks called *plexuses* after leaving the spinal cord

I believe I have a pinched nerve somewhere between L1 and S5. Boy, does that smart!

(Text continues on page 116.)

The spinal nerves

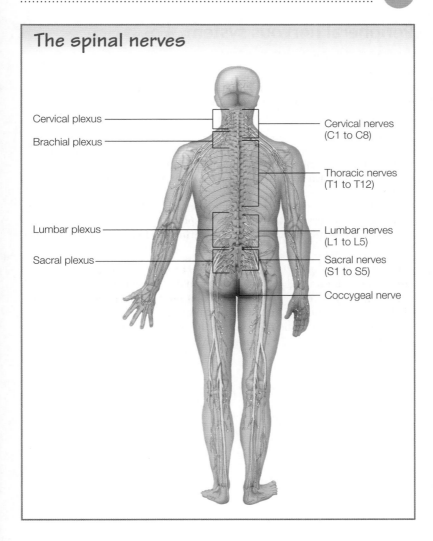

Cervical plexus

Brachial plexus

Lumbar plexus

Sacral plexus

Cervical nerves
(C1 to C8)

Thoracic nerves
(T1 to T12)

Lumbar nerves
(L1 to L5)

Sacral nerves
(S1 to S5)

Coccygeal nerve

Peripheral nervous system *(continued)*
Autonomic nervous system
- Innervates all internal organs
- Has two subdivisions: sympathetic and parasympathetic
- Divisions counterbalance each other's activities to keep body systems running smoothly

Sympathetic nervous system
- Composed of *preganglionic neurons* that exit the spinal cord between T1 and L2 and enter small ganglia near the cord
- The ganglia form a chain that spreads the impulse to *postganglionic neurons*
- Postganglionic neurons reach many organs and glands; can produce widespread, generalized physiologic responses
- Functions mainly during stress, triggering the fight-or-flight response

Parasympathetic nervous system
- Composed of fibers that leave the CNS by way of cranial nerves (from the midbrain and medulla) and spinal nerves (between S2 and S4)
- Each parasympathetic nerve has a long preganglionic fiber that travels to a ganglion near a particular organ or gland
- A short postganglionic fiber enters the organ or gland
- Creates a more specific response involving only one organ or gland

Autonomic nervous system

Effector organs	Parasympathetic responses	Sympathetic responses
Eye • Radial muscle of iris • Sphincter muscle of iris	• None • Contraction for near vision	• Contraction (mydriasis) • None
Heart	• Decreased rate and contractility	• Increased rate and contractility
Lung • Bronchial muscle	• Contraction	• Relaxation
Stomach • Motility and tone • Sphincters	• Increased • Relaxation	• Decreased (usually) • Contraction (usually)
Intestine • Motility and tone • Sphincters	• Increased • Relaxation	• Decreased • Contraction
Urinary bladder • Bladder muscle • Trigone and sphincter	• Contraction • Relaxation	• Relaxation • Contraction
Skin • Erector pili • Sweat glands	• None • Generalized secretion	• Contraction • Slight localized secretion
Adrenal medulla	• None	• Secretion of epinephrine and norepinephrine
Liver	• None	• Glycogenolysis
Pancreas • Acini	• Increased secretion	• Decreased secretion
Adipose tissue	• None	• Lipolysis
Juxtaglomerular cells	• None	• Increased renin secretion

Special sense organs

- Sensory receptors send messages to the brain to allow the body to interact with the environment
- The brain also receives stimulation from the special sense organs—the eyes, ears, and gustatory and olfactory organs

Eyes

- Are sensory organs for vision
- Consist of extraocular and intraocular structures

Extraocular structures

- *Bony orbits*: protect the eyes from trauma
- *Eyelids* (or *palpebrae*) and *eyelashes*: protect the eyes from injury, dust, and foreign bodies
- *Conjunctivae* (thin mucous membranes that line the inner surface of each eyelid and the anterior portion of the sclera): guard against invasion by foreign matter
- The structures of the *lacrimal apparatus* (*lacrimal glands*, *punctum*, *lacrimal sac*, and *nasolacrimal duct*): lubricate and protect the cornea and conjunctivae by producing and absorbing tears
- *Extraocular muscles*: hold the eyes in place and control movement, helping create binocular vision

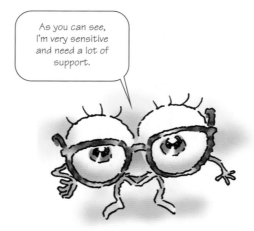

As you can see, I'm very sensitive and need a lot of support.

(Text continues on page 120.)

Extraocular structures

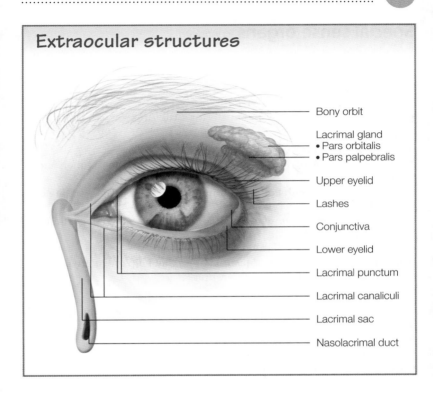

- Bony orbit
- Lacrimal gland
  - Pars orbitalis
  - Pars palpebralis
- Upper eyelid
- Lashes
- Conjunctiva
- Lower eyelid
- Lacrimal punctum
- Lacrimal canaliculi
- Lacrimal sac
- Nasolacrimal duct

Special sense organs *(continued)*

Eyes *(continued)*

Intraocular structures

- Contained within the eyeball
- Are directly involved with vision
- Are divided into anterior and posterior structures

Anterior structures

- *Sclera*: maintains the eyeball's size and form
- *Cornea*: a smooth, transparent tissue; highly sensitive to touch and is kept moist by tears
- *Iris*: contains smooth and radial muscles; has an opening in the center for the *pupil,* which regulates light entry
- *Anterior* and *posterior chambers*: filled with a clear, watery fluid called *aqueous humor*
- *Lens*: refracts and focuses light onto the retina
- *Ciliary body*: controls the lens thickness and helps regulate the light focused through the lens onto the retina

Posterior structures

- *Vitreous humor*: maintains placement of the retina and the spherical shape of the eyeball
- *Posterior sclera*: covers the optic nerve
- *Choroid*: contains many small arteries and veins
- *Retina*: receives visual stimuli and sends them to the brain

(Text continues on page 122.)

Intraocular structures

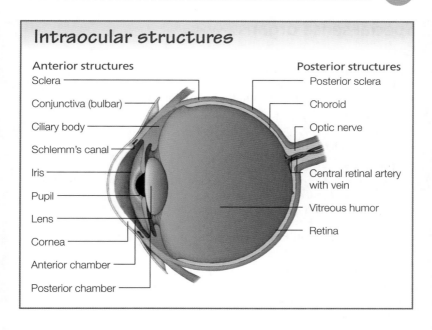

Anterior structures

Sclera

Conjunctiva (bulbar)

Ciliary body

Schlemm's canal

Iris

Pupil

Lens

Cornea

Anterior chamber

Posterior chamber

Posterior structures

Posterior sclera

Choroid

Optic nerve

Central retinal artery with vein

Vitreous humor

Retina

Special sense organs *(continued)*

Ears

- Are the organs of hearing
- Maintain the body's equilibrium
- Divided into the external, middle, and inner ear

External ear structures
- Consist of the *auricle* (pinna) and the *external auditory canal*
- Serve to collect sound

Middle ear structures
- *Tympanic membrane*: transmits sound vibrations to the internal ear
- *Eustachian tube*: equalizes pressure within the ear
- *Oval window* and *round window*: transmit vibrations to the inner ear
- *Malleus, incus,* and *stapes*: conduct vibratory motion of the tympanum to the oval window

Inner ear structures
- Contain the *vestibule, cochlea,* and *semicircular canals*
- Receive vibrations from the middle ear that stimulate nerve impulses
- Impulses travel to the brain, and the cerebral cortex interprets the sound

(Text continues on page 124.)

Ear structures

External ear **Middle ear** **Inner ear**

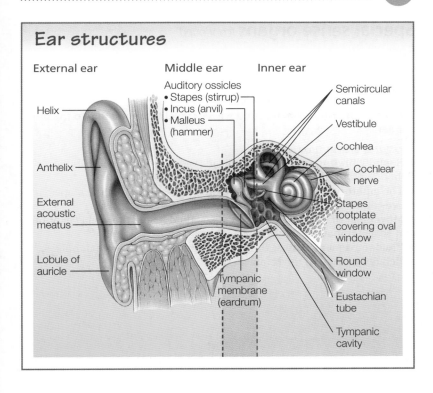

External ear:
- Helix
- Anthelix
- External acoustic meatus
- Lobule of auricle

Middle ear:
- Auditory ossicles
  - Stapes (stirrup)
  - Incus (anvil)
  - Malleus (hammer)
- Tympanic membrane (eardrum)

Inner ear:
- Semicircular canals
- Vestibule
- Cochlea
- Cochlear nerve
- Stapes footplate covering oval window
- Round window
- Eustachian tube
- Tympanic cavity

Special sense organs *(continued)*

Ears *(continued)*

Hearing pathways

- *Air conduction*: when sound waves travel in the air through the external and middle ear to the inner ear
- *Bone conduction*: when sound waves travel through bone to the inner ear

Sound transmission

- Sound vibrations strike the eardrum (see #1 in the illustration at right)
- The auditory ossicles then vibrate and the footplate of the stapes moves at the oval window (#2)
- Movement of the oval window causes fluid inside the scala vestibuli and scala tympani to move (#3)
- Fluid movement against the cochlear duct sets off nerve impulses, which are carried to the brain via the cochlear nerve (#4)

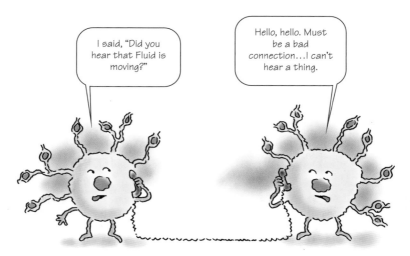

(Text continues on page 126.)

Sound transmission

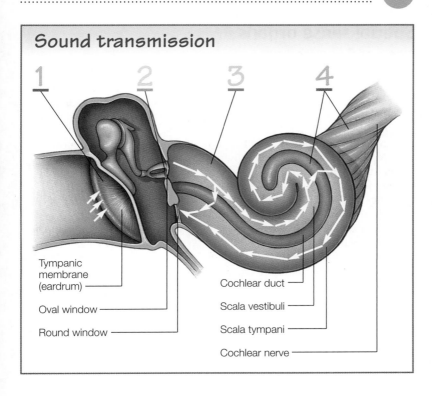

1

2

3

4

Tympanic membrane (eardrum)

Oval window

Round window

Cochlear duct

Scala vestibuli

Scala tympani

Cochlear nerve

Special sense organs *(continued)*
Nose and mouth

- The nose is the sense organ for smell
    - Receptors for fibers of the olfactory nerve (CN I) reside in the mucosal epithelium (lining the uppermost portion of the nasal cavity)
    - Receptors, consisting of hair cells, are called *olfactory* (smell) *receptors*
    - Receptors are highly sensitive, stimulated by the slightest odor
    - Receptors are also easily fatigued and stop sensing even strong smells after a short time
- The mouth contains receptors for taste nerve fibers (located in branches of CNs VII and IX); most reside on the tongue and roof of the mouth
    - Receptors are called *taste buds*; most sit on raised protrusions of the skin surface called *papillae*
    - Taste buds are stimulated by chemicals and respond to four taste sensations: sweet, sour, bitter, and salty
    - All the other flavor sensations result from a combination of olfactory-receptor and taste-bud stimulation

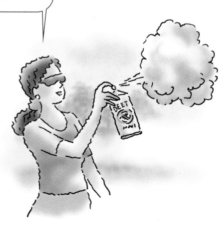

For certain odors, the time it takes my olfactory receptors to tire out takes way too long.

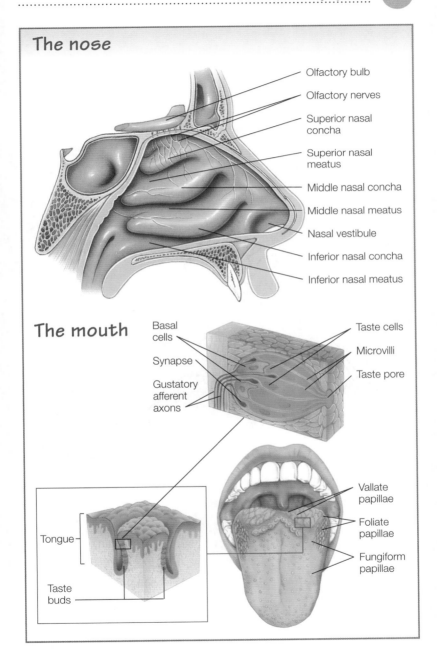

The nose

- Olfactory bulb
- Olfactory nerves
- Superior nasal concha
- Superior nasal meatus
- Middle nasal concha
- Middle nasal meatus
- Nasal vestibule
- Inferior nasal concha
- Inferior nasal meatus

The mouth

- Basal cells
- Synapse
- Gustatory afferent axons
- Taste cells
- Microvilli
- Taste pore

- Tongue
- Taste buds

- Vallate papillae
- Foliate papillae
- Fungiform papillae

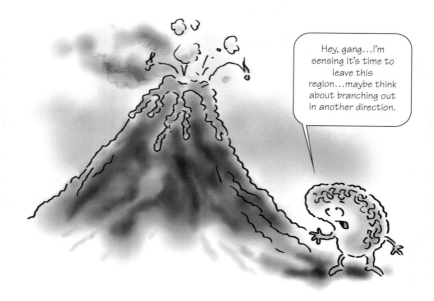

7

Endocrine system

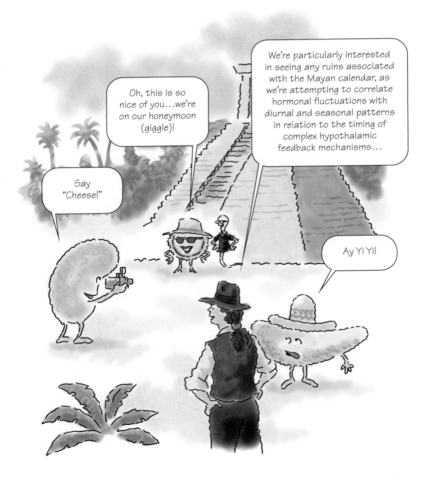

Endocrine system basics

- Helps regulate and integrate the body's metabolic activities (along with the nervous system)
- Consists of three major components: glands, hormones, and receptors

Glands

- Composed of specialized cell clusters or organs
- Secrete hormones directly into the bloodstream to regulate body function
- Major glands are the pituitary gland, thyroid gland, parathyroid gland, adrenal glands, pancreas, thymus, pineal gland, and gonads (ovaries and testes)

> Glands are specialized cell clusters, or organs, that secrete hormones directly into the bloodstream.

(Text continues on page 132.)

Components of the endocrine system

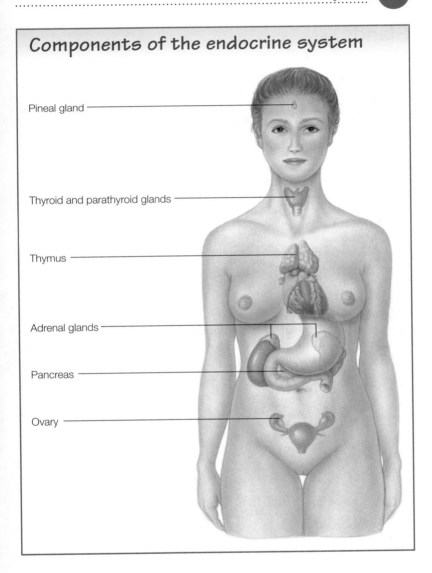

Pineal gland

Thyroid and parathyroid glands

Thymus

Adrenal glands

Pancreas

Ovary

Glands *(continued)*

Pituitary gland

- A pea-sized gland that rests in the *sella turcica* (a depression in the sphenoid bone at the base of the brain)
- Connects with the hypothalamus via the infundibulum, from which it receives chemical and nervous stimulation
- Composed of two main regions: anterior and posterior

Anterior pituitary
- Also known as adenohypophysis
- Larger of the two regions
- Produces at least six hormones:
  - Growth hormone (GH), or somatotropin
  - Thyroid-stimulating hormone (TSH), or thyrotropin
  - Corticotropin
  - Follicle-stimulating hormone (FSH)
  - Luteinizing hormone (LH)
  - Prolactin

Posterior pituitary
- Makes up about 25% of the gland
- Serves as a storage area for antidiuretic hormone (ADH), also known as vasopressin, and oxytocin, which are produced by the hypothalamus

(Text continues on page 134.)

Pituitary gland

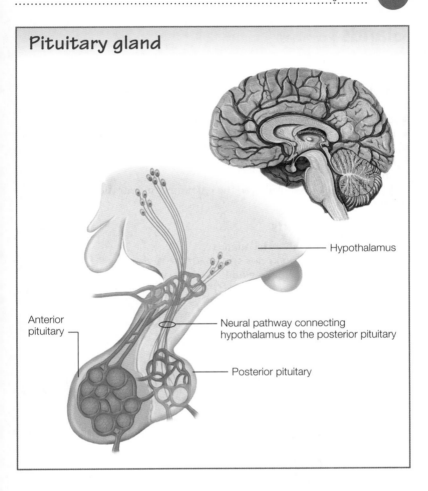

Hypothalamus

Anterior pituitary

Neural pathway connecting hypothalamus to the posterior pituitary

Posterior pituitary

Glands (continued)

Thyroid gland

- Has two lobes that function as one unit
- Produces the hormones *thyroxine* (T_4) and *triiodothyronine* (T_3)
- Collectively referred to as thyroid hormone
- Considered the body's major metabolic hormone
- Regulates metabolism by speeding cellular respiration
- Also produces calcitonin
- Maintains blood calcium level by inhibiting the release of calcium from the bone
- Alters secretion according to the calcium concentration in surrounding fluid

Parathyroid glands

- Smallest known endocrine glands
- Embedded on the posterior surface of the thyroid
- Work together as a single gland
- Produce *parathyroid hormone* (PTH), which helps regulate blood's calcium balance

> Although it's in my throat, the thyroid gland is really near and dear to my heart. It secretes calcitonin to inhibit the release of calcium from bone, which helps keep me strong and healthy.

(Text continues on page 136.)

Thyroid and parathyroid glands

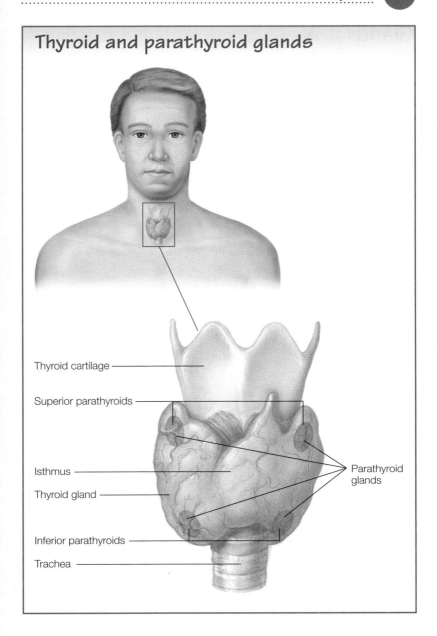

Thyroid cartilage

Superior parathyroids

Isthmus

Thyroid gland

Inferior parathyroids

Trachea

Parathyroid glands

Glands *(continued)*

Adrenal glands

- Consist of two almond-shaped glands, each lying on top of a kidney
- Contain two distinct structures: the *adrenal cortex* and the *adrenal medulla*
- Each function as separate endocrine glands

Adrenal cortex

- Forms the bulk of the adrenal gland
- Has three zones, or cell layers
  - *Zona glomerulosa*: produces mineralocorticoids (primarily aldosterone)
  - *Zona fasciculata*: produces glucocorticoids (cortisol [hydrocortisone], cortisone, and corticosterone) and small amounts of androgen and estrogen
  - *Zona reticularis*: produces some sex hormones

Adrenal medulla

- Functions as part of the sympathetic nervous system
- Produces two catecholamines: epinephrine and norepinephrine
- Considered a neuroendocrine structure

(Text continues on page 138.)

Adrenal glands

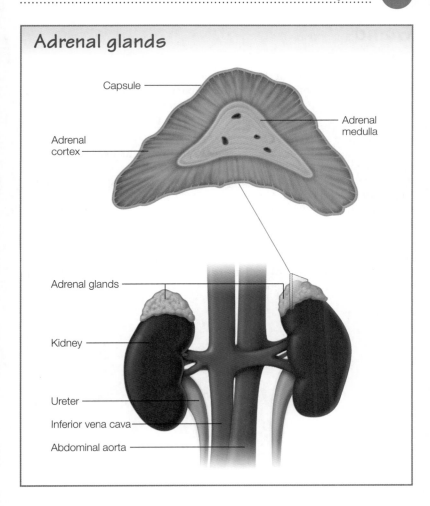

Glands *(continued)*

Pancreas

- Nestled in the curve of the duodenum
- Stretches horizontally behind the stomach and extends to the spleen
- Performs both *endocrine* and *exocrine* functions

Endocrine functions

- Regulated by *islet cells*, or *islets of Langerhans*
- Alpha cells produce *glucagon* (raises the blood glucose level by triggering the breakdown of glycogen to glucose)
- Beta cells produce *insulin* (lowers the blood glucose level by stimulating the conversion of glucose to glycogen)
- Delta cells produce *somatostatin* (inhibits the release of GH, corticotropin, and certain other hormones)

Exocrine functions

- Regulated by *acinar cells* (which make up most of the pancreas)
- Involves secretion of digestive enzymes (which flow through the pancreatic duct to the duodenum)

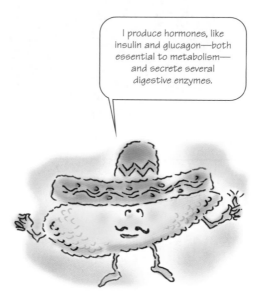

I produce hormones, like insulin and glucagon—both essential to metabolism—and secrete several digestive enzymes.

(Text continues on page 140.)

Pancreas

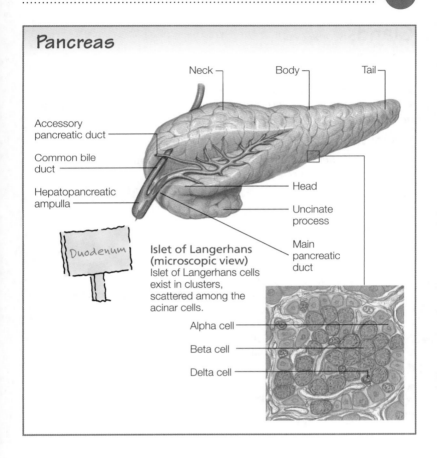

Neck

Body

Tail

Accessory
pancreatic duct

Common bile
duct

Hepatopancreatic
ampulla

Duodenum

Head

Uncinate
process

Main
pancreatic
duct

**Islet of Langerhans
(microscopic view)**
Islet of Langerhans cells
exist in clusters,
scattered among the
acinar cells.

Alpha cell

Beta cell

Delta cell

Glands (continued)

Thymus

- Contains lymphatic tissue
- Produces T cells (important in cell-mediated immunity)
- Produces the peptide hormones *thymosin* and *thymopoietin* (promote growth of peripheral lymphoid tissue)

Pineal gland

- Lies at the back of the third ventricle of the brain
- Produces the hormone *melatonin*

Gonads

- Includes the ovaries in females
- Includes the testes in males

Ovaries

- Produce ova (eggs)
- Produce estrogen and progesterone
  - Promote development and maintenance of female sex characteristics
  - Regulate the menstrual cycle
  - Maintain the uterus for pregnancy
  - Help prepare the mammary glands for lactation

Testes

- Produce spermatozoa
- Produce testosterone, which stimulates and maintains masculine sex characteristics and triggers the male sex drive

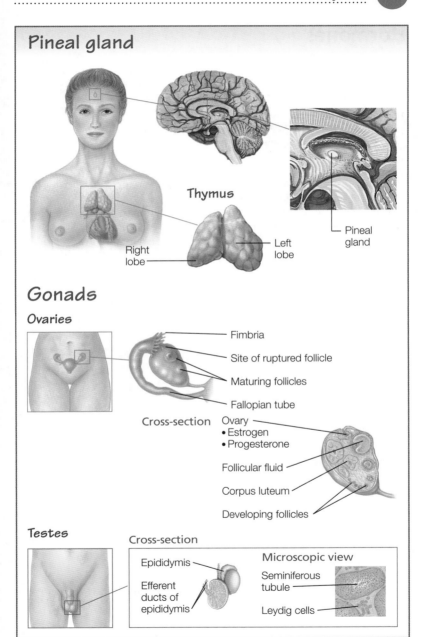

Pineal gland

Thymus

Right lobe — Left lobe

Pineal gland

Gonads

Ovaries

Fimbria

Site of ruptured follicle

Maturing follicles

Fallopian tube

Cross-section Ovary
• Estrogen
• Progesterone

Follicular fluid

Corpus luteum

Developing follicles

Testes

Cross-section

Epididymis

Efferent ducts of epididymis

Microscopic view

Seminiferous tubule

Leydig cells

Hormones

- Chemical substances secreted by glands in response to stimulation
- Trigger or regulate the activity of an organ or a group of cells

Hormonal release and transport

- Hormone release patterns vary greatly
  - Corticotropin and cortisol are released in spurts in response to body rhythm cycles; levels of these hormones peak in the morning
  - Secretion of PTH and prolactin occurs fairly evenly throughout the day
  - Secretion of insulin can occur at a steady rate or sporadically, depending on blood glucose levels
- When a hormone reaches its target site, it binds to a specific receptor on the cell membrane or within the cell
- After binding occurs, each hormone produces unique physiologic changes, depending on its target site and its specific action at that site
- A particular hormone may have different effects at different target sites

(Text continues on page 144.)

Classification of hormones

Hormones are classified by their molecular structure as polypeptides, steroids, or amines.

Classification	Hormones
Polypeptides Made of many amino acids connected by peptide bonds	• Anterior pituitary hormones (GH, TSH, FSH, LH, and prolactin) • Posterior pituitary hormones (ADH and oxytocin) • Parathyroid hormone (PTH) • Pancreatic hormones (insulin and glucagon)
Steroids Derived from cholesterol	• Adrenocortical hormones (aldosterone and cortisol) • Sex hormones (estrogen and progesterone in females and testosterone in males)
Amines Derived from tyrosine	• Thyroid hormones (T_4 and T_3) • Catecholamines (epinephrine, norepinephrine, and dopamine)

Hormones *(continued)*

Hormonal regulation

- A feedback mechanism regulates hormone production and secretion to maintain the body's delicate equilibrium
- The mechanism involves hormones, blood chemicals and metabolites, and the nervous system
- System can be simple or complex

Simple feedback

- When the level of one substance regulates the secretion of hormones
- Example: a low serum calcium level stimulates the parathyroid gland to release PTH

Complex feedback

- Triggered by hypothalamic stimulation
- First, the hypothalamus sends releasing and inhibiting factors or hormones to the anterior pituitary
- The anterior pituitary responds by secreting *tropic hormones* (GH, PRL, corticotropin, TSH, FSH, and LH)
- These hormones stimulate the target organ to release other hormones that regulate various body functions
- When these hormones reach normal levels, a feedback mechanism inhibits further hypothalamic and pituitary secretion

Receptors

- Protein molecules that bind specifically with other molecules (such as hormones) to trigger specific physiologic changes in a target cell
- Sensitivity of a target cell depends on how many receptors it has for a hormone
- The more receptor sites, the more sensitive the target cell

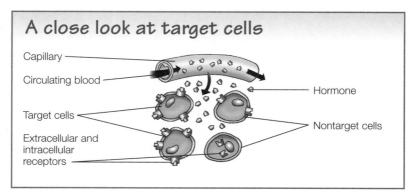

A close look at target cells

Capillary

Circulating blood

Hormone

Target cells

Nontarget cells

Extracellular and intracellular receptors

The feedback loop

This diagram shows the negative feedback mechanism that helps regulate the endocrine system.

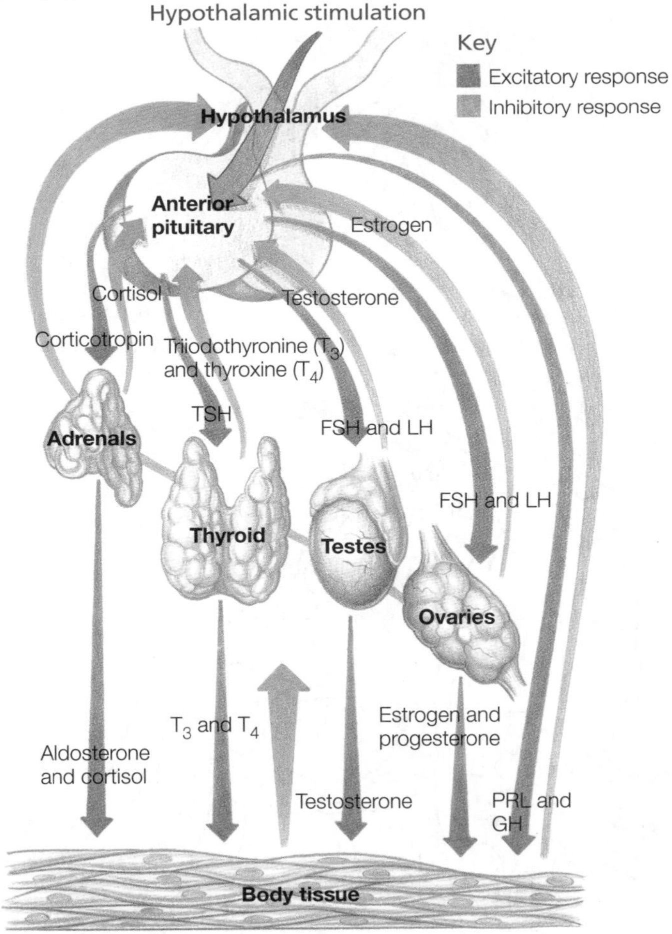

Hypothalamic stimulation

Key
■ Excitatory response
■ Inhibitory response

Hypothalamus

Anterior pituitary

Estrogen

Cortisol

Testosterone

Corticotropin

Triiodothyronine (T_3) and thyroxine (T_4)

TSH

FSH and LH

Adrenals

FSH and LH

Thyroid

Testes

Ovaries

T_3 and T_4

Estrogen and progesterone

Aldosterone and cortisol

Testosterone

PRL and GH

Body tissue

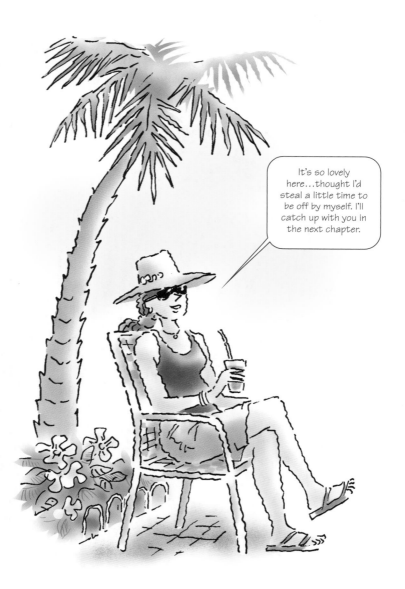

8
Cardiovascular system

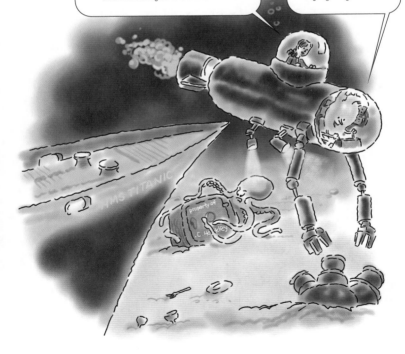

Cardiovascular system basics

- Consists of the heart, blood vessels, and lymphatics
- Brings life-sustaining oxygen and nutrients to the body's cells
- Removes metabolic waste products
- Carries hormones from one part of the body to another

The heart

- Is about the size of a closed fist
- Lies beneath the sternum in the mediastinum (the cavity between the lungs), between the second and sixth ribs
- Rests obliquely, with its right side below and almost in front of the left, making its broad part or top at its upper right, and its pointed end (apex) at its lower left
- Produces the loudest heart sounds (the point of maximal impulse) at the apex
- Consists of two separate pumps:
  - The right side pumps the blood to the lungs to receive oxygen
  - The left side pumps the oxygenated blood to the rest of the body

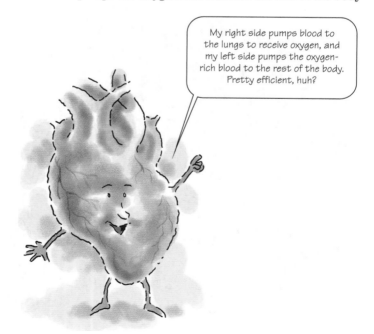

My right side pumps blood to the lungs to receive oxygen, and my left side pumps the oxygen-rich blood to the rest of the body. Pretty efficient, huh?

(Text continues on page 150.)

Location of the heart

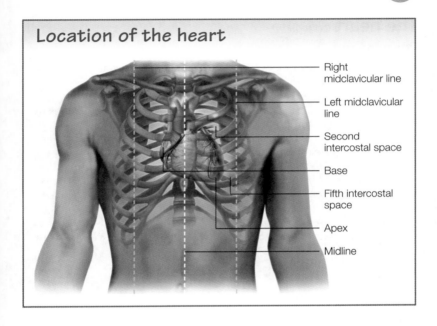

Right midclavicular line

Left midclavicular line

Second intercostal space

Base

Fifth intercostal space

Apex

Midline

The heart *(continued)*

Pericardium

- Consists of a fibroserous sac that surrounds the heart and the roots of the *great vessels*
- Composed of two layers:
  - The *fibrous pericardium* (tough, white fibrous tissue) fits loosely around the heart, protecting it
  - The *serous pericardium* is a thin, smooth inner portion
- The serous pericardium also has two layers:
  - The *parietal layer* lines the inside of the fibrous pericardium
  - The *visceral layer* adheres to the surface of the heart
- Residing between the fibrous and serous pericardium is the *pericardial space*
  - Contains *pericardial fluid*
  - Fluid lubricates the space and allows the heart to move easily during contraction

Heart wall

- Consists of three layers
- *Epicardium*: outer layer that's made up of squamous epithelial cells overlying connective tissue
- *Myocardium*: middle layer that forms most of the heart wall; it has striated muscle fibers that cause the heart to contract
- *Endocardium*: inner layer that consists of endothelial tissue with small blood vessels and bundles of smooth muscle

(Text continues on page 152.)

The pericardium

Anterior view

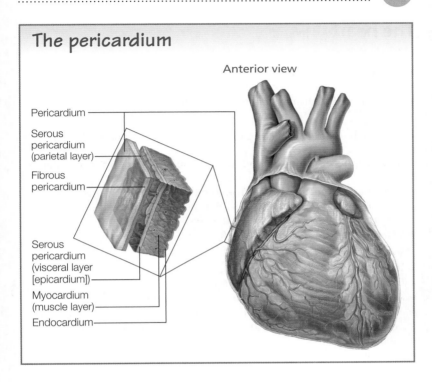

Pericardium

Serous pericardium (parietal layer)

Fibrous pericardium

Serous pericardium (visceral layer [epicardium])

Myocardium (muscle layer)

Endocardium

The heart *(continued)*

Heart chambers

- Consists of four hollow chambers
- Two *atria* (singular: *atrium*) form the upper chambers
- Two *ventricles* form the lower chambers

Atria

- Receive blood returning to the heart and supply blood to the ventricles
- *Right atrium*: receives blood from the superior and inferior venae cavae
- *Left atrium*: receives blood from the two pulmonary veins
  - Smaller but has thicker walls than the right atrium
  - Forms the uppermost part of the heart's left border
- Separated by the *interatrial septum*

Ventricles

- Receive blood from the atria
- Composed of highly developed musculature
- Are larger and have thicker walls than the atria
- *Right ventricle*: pumps blood to the lungs
- *Left ventricle*: larger than the right; pumps blood through all other vessels of the body
- Separated by the *interventricular septum*

(Text continues on page 154.)

Inside the heart

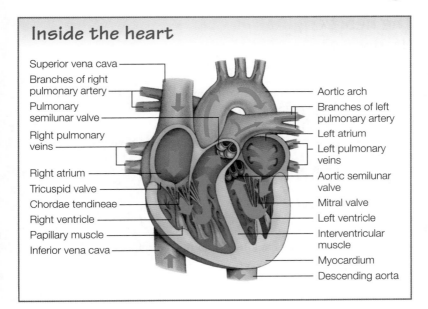

Superior vena cava

Branches of right pulmonary artery

Pulmonary semilunar valve

Right pulmonary veins

Right atrium

Tricuspid valve

Chordae tendineae

Right ventricle

Papillary muscle

Inferior vena cava

Aortic arch

Branches of left pulmonary artery

Left atrium

Left pulmonary veins

Aortic semilunar valve

Mitral valve

Left ventricle

Interventricular muscle

Myocardium

Descending aorta

The heart *(continued)*

Heart valves

- Allow forward flow of blood through the heart and prevent backward flow
- Open and close in response to pressure changes within the heart
- Consists of four valves: two *AV valves* and two *semilunar valves*

AV valves

- *Tricuspid valve*: prevents backflow from the right ventricle into the right atrium
- *Mitral valve:* prevents backflow from the left ventricle into the left atrium

Semilunar valves

- *Pulmonic valve*: prevents backflow from the pulmonary artery into the right ventricle
- *Aortic valve*: prevents backflow from the aorta into the left ventricle

Valve cusps

- The tricuspid valve has three triangular *cusps,* or leaflets
- The mitral valve (*bicuspid valve*) contains two cusps
- *Chordae tendineae* attach the cusps of the AV valves to papillary muscles in the ventricles
- The semilunar valves have three cusps that are shaped like half-moons

(Text continues on page 156.)

Heart valves

Top View

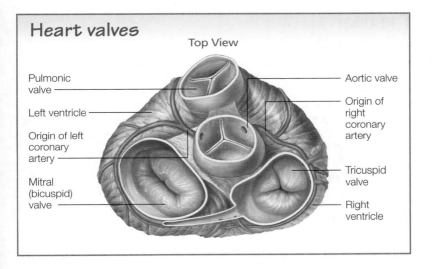

Pulmonic valve

Left ventricle

Origin of left coronary artery

Mitral (bicuspid) valve

Aortic valve

Origin of right coronary artery

Tricuspid valve

Right ventricle

The heart (continued)

Cardiac conduction system

● Contains *pacemaker cells*, which have three unique characteristics:
  – *Automaticity*: the ability to generate an electrical impulse automatically
  – *Conductivity*: the ability to pass the impulse to the next cell
  – *Contractility*: the ability to shorten the heart fibers when receiving the impulse
● Normal pacemaker is the *SA node*
  – Generates an impulse of 60 to 100 times/minute
  – Spreads an impulse throughout the right and left atria, resulting in *atrial contraction*
● The *AV node* slows impulse conduction between the atria and ventricles, allowing time for the contracting atria to fill the ventricles with blood
● From the AV node, the impulse travels to the *bundle of His*, then along the *bundle branches* and, finally down the *Purkinje fibers*, resulting in *ventricular contraction*
● If the SA node fails to fire, the AV node will generate an impulse of 40 to 60 times/minute
● If the SA node and AV node fail, the ventricles can generate their own impulse of 20 to 40 times/minute

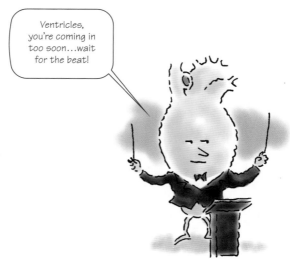

(Text continues on page 158.)

Cardiac conduction

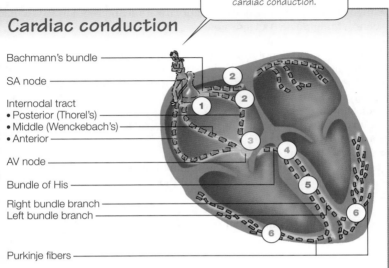

The firing of the SA node sets off a chain reaction in cardiac conduction.

Bachmann's bundle

SA node

Internodal tract
• Posterior (Thorel's)
• Middle (Wenckebach's)
• Anterior

AV node

Bundle of His

Right bundle branch
Left bundle branch

Purkinje fibers

The heart *(continued)*

The depolarization-repolarization cycle

● Involves cycles of cardiac cell depolarization and repolarization that occur with impulse transmission
● Incorporates five phases
● *Phase 0*: Rapid depolarization, in which sodium and calcium move rapidly into the cell
● *Phase 1*: Early repolarization, in which sodium channels close
● *Phase 2*: Plateau phase, in which calcium continues to flow in and potassium flows out of the cell
● *Phase 3*: Rapid depolarization, in which calcium channels close and potassium flows out rapidly
● *Phase 4*: Resting phase
  – Active transport through the sodium-potassium pump begins restoring potassium to the inside of the cell and sodium to the outside
  – The cell membrane becomes impermeable to sodium
  – Potassium may move out of the cell

(Text continues on page 160.)

Depolarization-repolarization cycle

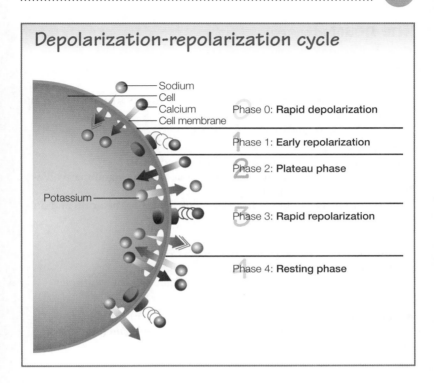

Sodium
Cell
Calcium
Cell membrane

Potassium

Phase 0: **Rapid depolarization**

Phase 1: **Early repolarization**

Phase 2: **Plateau phase**

Phase 3: **Rapid repolarization**

Phase 4: **Resting phase**

The heart *(continued)*

Cardiac cycle

- Involves the period from the beginning of one heartbeat to the beginning of the next
- Requires precise electrical and mechanical events to ensure adequate cardiac output
- Consists of two phases: *systole* and *diastole*

Systole

- Period in which ventricular contraction occurs
- The AV valves (mitral and tricuspid) close and the semilunar valves (pulmonic and aortic) open
- The ventricles eject blood from the ventricles into the aorta and pulmonary artery

Diastole

- Semilunar valves close and the AV valves open
- Blood flows into the ventricles from the atria
- The atria contract to send the remaining blood to the ventricles

Cardiac output

- Refers to the amount of blood the heart pumps in 1 minute
- Equals the heart rate multiplied by the *stroke volume* (amount of blood ejected with each heartbeat)

(Text continues on page 162.)

Events in the cardiac cycle

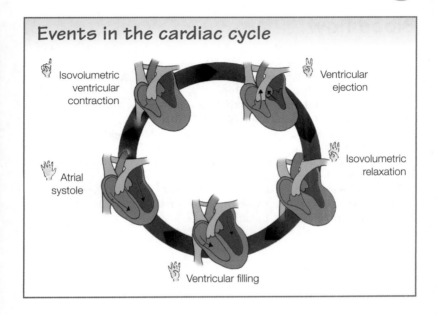

Isovolumetric ventricular contraction

Ventricular ejection

Isovolumetric relaxation

Atrial systole

Ventricular filling

Blood flow

● Five distinct types of blood vessels carry blood through the vascular system: *arteries, arterioles, capillaries, venules,* and *veins*

● *Arteries*: have thick, muscular walls to accommodate the flow of blood at high speeds and pressures

● *Arterioles*: have thinner walls than arteries; they constrict or dilate to control blood flow to the capillaries

● *Capillaries*: microscopic vessels with walls composed of a single layer of endothelial cells

● *Venules*: gather blood from capillaries; their walls are thinner than those of arterioles

● *Veins*: have thinner walls than arteries but have larger diameters because of the low blood pressures of venous return to the heart; valves in the veins prevent blood backflow

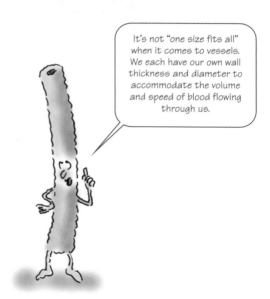

It's not "one size fits all" when it comes to vessels. We each have our own wall thickness and diameter to accommodate the volume and speed of blood flowing through us.

(Text continues on page 164.)

Arteriovenous circulation

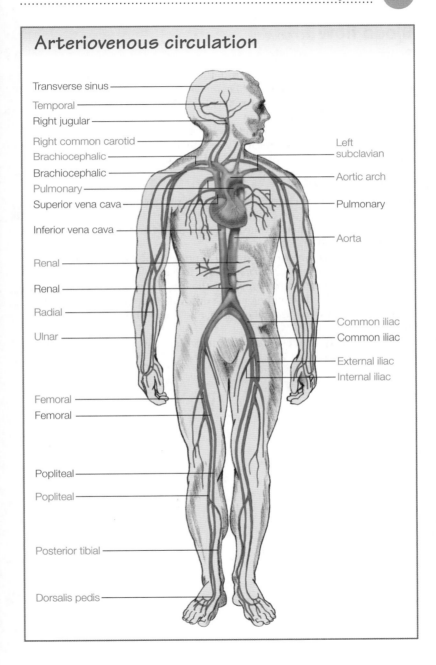

Transverse sinus

Temporal

Right jugular

Right common carotid

Brachiocephalic

Brachiocephalic

Pulmonary

Superior vena cava

Inferior vena cava

Renal

Renal

Radial

Ulnar

Femoral

Femoral

Popliteal

Popliteal

Posterior tibial

Dorsalis pedis

Left subclavian

Aortic arch

Pulmonary

Aorta

Common iliac

Common iliac

External iliac

Internal iliac

Blood flow *(continued)*

Pulmonary circulation

- Unoxygenated blood travels from the right ventricle through the pulmonic valve into the *pulmonary arteries*
- Blood passes through progressively smaller arteries and arterioles into the capillaries of the lungs
- Blood reaches the *alveoli* and exchanges carbon dioxide for oxygen
- Oxygenated blood then returns via venules and veins to the *pulmonary veins*, which carry it back to the left atrium

Systemic circulation

- The aorta branches into vessels that supply specific organs and areas of the body
- Three arteries branch off the top of the aortic arch to supply the upper body with blood:
    - The *left common carotid artery* supplies blood to the brain
    - The *left subclavian artery* supplies the arms
    - The *innominate artery* supplies the upper chest
- Branches of the descending aorta supply the organs of the GI and genitourinary systems, spinal column, and lower chest and abdominal muscles
- Then the aorta divides into the *iliac arteries*, which further divide into *femoral arteries*

(Text continues on page 166.)

Blood circulation

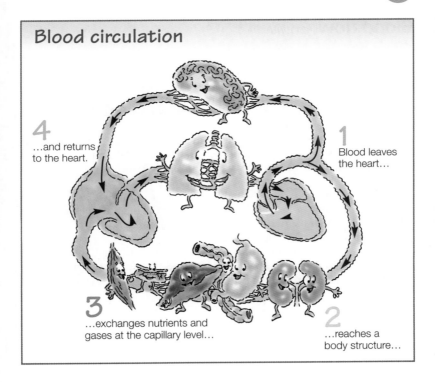

4 ...and returns to the heart.

1 Blood leaves the heart...

3 ...exchanges nutrients and gases at the capillary level...

2 ...reaches a body structure...

Blood flow *(continued)*

Coronary circulation

- Coronary arteries and their branches supply the heart with oxygenated blood
- Cardiac veins remove oxygen-depleted blood
- During systole, blood is ejected into the aorta from the left ventricle
- During diastole, blood flows out of the heart and then through the coronary arteries to nourish the heart muscle
- The *right coronary artery* supplies blood to the right atrium, part of the left atrium, most of the right ventricle, and the inferior part of the left ventricle
- The *left coronary artery*, which splits into the *anterior descending artery* and *circumflex artery*, supplies blood to the left atrium, most of the left ventricle, and most of the interventricular septum
- The *cardiac veins* lie superficial to the arteries
- The largest vein, the *coronary sinus*, opens into the right atrium
- Most of the major cardiac veins empty into the coronary sinus, except for the *anterior cardiac veins*, which empty into the right atrium

Coronary arteries

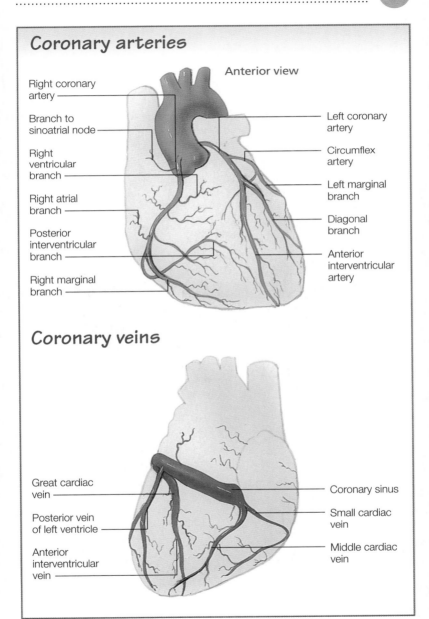

Anterior view

Right coronary artery

Branch to sinoatrial node

Right ventricular branch

Right atrial branch

Posterior interventricular branch

Right marginal branch

Left coronary artery

Circumflex artery

Left marginal branch

Diagonal branch

Anterior interventricular artery

Coronary veins

Great cardiac vein

Posterior vein of left ventricle

Anterior interventricular vein

Coronary sinus

Small cardiac vein

Middle cardiac vein

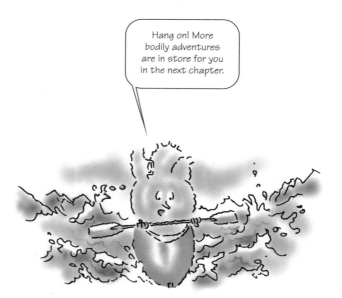

9
Hematologic system

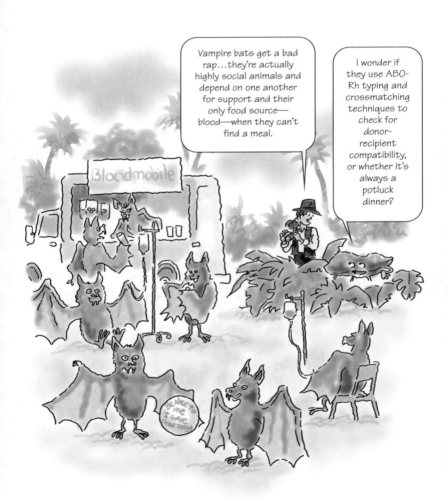

Hematologic system basics

- Consists of the blood and bone marrow
- Uses blood to deliver oxygen and nutrients to all tissues, remove wastes, and transport gases, blood cells, immune cells, and hormones throughout the body
- Manufactures new blood cells through a process called *hematopoiesis*
- Uses *multipotential stem cells* in bone marrow to give rise to five distinct cell types, called *unipotential stem cells*
- Causes unipotential cells to differentiate into one of four types of blood cells: erythrocytes (the most common type), granulocytes, agranulocytes, or platelets

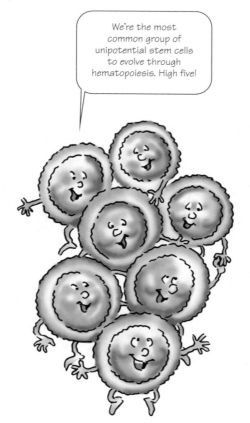

We're the most common group of unipotential stem cells to evolve through hematopoiesis. High five!

(Text continues on page 172.)

The development of blood cells

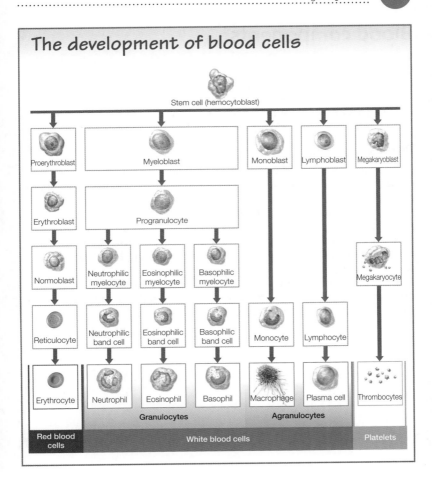

Blood components

- Consists of various formed elements (*blood cells*) suspended in a fluid (*plasma*)
- Contains the following formed elements:
  - red blood cells (RBCs), or erythrocytes
  - white blood cells (WBCs), or leukocytes
  - platelets, or thrombocytes

Red blood cells

- Transport oxygen and carbon dioxide to and from body tissues
- Contain *hemoglobin*, the oxygen-carrying substance that gives blood its red color
- Have an average life span of 120 days
- Begin in the bone marrow, which releases RBCs into circulation in immature form as *reticulocytes*; these mature into RBCs in about 1 day
- Are removed from circulation by the spleen when they become old and worn out
- Are replenished during periods of depletion (for example, with hemorrhage) by the bone marrow, which increases reticulocyte production to maintain the normal RBC count

(*Text continues on page 174.*)

Blood components

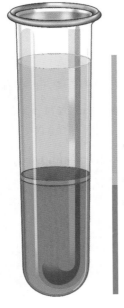

- Plasma (55%)

- White blood cells (WBCs) and platelets (< 1%)
- Red blood cells (RBCs) (45%)

Here's a breakdown of formed elements in the blood.

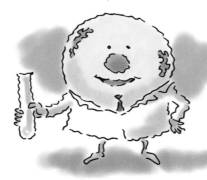

Blood components *(continued)*
White blood cells
- Protect the body against harmful bacteria and infection
- Classified as *granulocytes* or *agranulocytes*

  ### Granulocytes
- Consist mostly of *neutrophils*, which account for 50% to 75% of circulating WBCs
- Consist also of *eosinophils*, which account for 0.3% to 7% of circulating WBCs
- Include *basophils*, which usually constitute fewer than 2% of circulating WBCs

  ### Agranulocytes
- Include *monocytes*, the largest of the WBCs, which constitute only 1% to 9% of WBCs in circulation
- Consist also of *lymphocytes*, the smallest of the WBCs and the second most numerous (20% to 43%)

Platelets
- Are small, colorless, disk-shaped cytoplasmic fragments split from cells in bone marrow called *megakaryocytes*
- Have a life span of approximately 10 days
- Perform three vital functions:
  - initiate contraction of damaged blood vessels to minimize blood loss
  - form *hemostatic plugs* in injured blood vessels
  - provide materials (along with plasma) that accelerate blood coagulation

(Text continues on page 176.)

White blood cells

Granulocytes (Contain a single multilobular nucleus and granules in the cytoplasm)			Agranulocytes (Lack specific cytoplasmic granules and have a nucleus without lobes)	
Neutrophils	*Eosinophils*	*Basophils*	*Monocytes*	*Lymphocytes*
• Engulf, ingest, and digest foreign materials (phagocytosis) • Worn-out neutrophils form the main component of pus	• Migrate from the bloodstream as a response to an allergic reaction • Defend against parasites and fight lung and skin infections	• Possess little or no phagocytic ability • May release heparin and histamine into blood and participate in delayed allergic reactions	• Devour invading organisms by phagocytosis • Migrate to tissue where they develop into macrophages, which participate in immunity 	• Derive from stem cells in the bone marrow • Consist of two types: – T lymphocytes, which directly attack an infected cell – B lymphocytes, which produce antibodies against specific antigens

Blood clotting

- Known as *hemostasis*, the complex process by which *platelets, plasma*, and *coagulation factors* interact to control bleeding
- Begins when a blood vessel ruptures and local *vasoconstriction* (decrease in the caliber of blood vessels) occurs to decrease blood flow to the area
- Continues as platelets and clotting factors become activated when exposed to the collagen layer of the damaged blood vessel
- Causes platelets to clump together (aggregate) by binding to the collagen, forming a loose platelet plug
- Results in a temporary seal and a site for clotting to take place

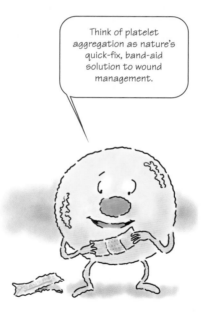

Think of platelet aggregation as nature's quick-fix, band-aid solution to wound management.

(Text continues on page 178.)

Blood clot formation

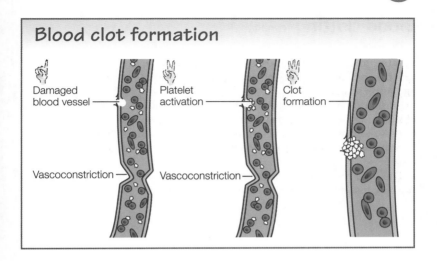

Blood clotting *(continued)*

Clotting pathway

● After creating a temporary clot, the damaged cells release tissue factor (*thromboplastin*), which activates the *extrinsic pathway* of the coagulation system

● Formation of a more stable clot requires initiation of the complex clotting mechanisms known as the *intrinsic pathway*

● This clotting system is activated by a protein, called factor XII, one of 12 substances necessary for coagulation and derived from plasma and tissue

● The final result of coagulation is a *fibrin clot*, an accumulation of a fibrous, insoluble protein at the site of the injury

(Text continues on page 180.)

How blood clots

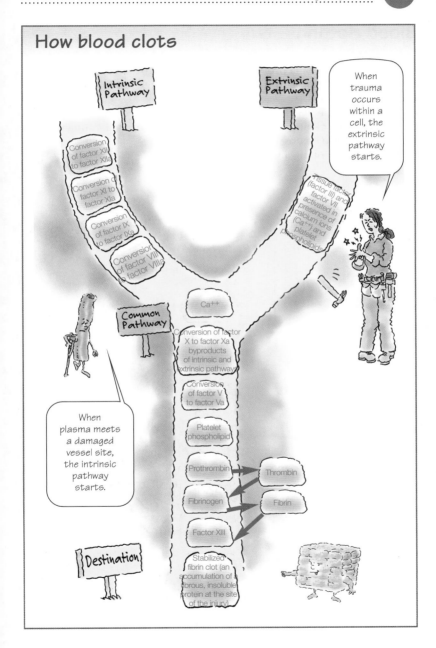

Blood clotting *(continued)*

Coagulation factors

- Composed of plasma proteins – except for factor IV (calcium), which is a mineral, and factor III (thromboplastin), which is a lipoprotein released from tissue
- Produced in the liver
- Activated in a chain reaction, with each one in turn activating the next factor in the chain
- Designated by name and Roman numeral

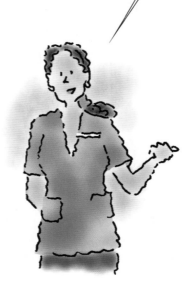

Clotting occurs through a chain reaction involving coagulation factors I through XIII. The Roman numeral designation refers to their order of discovery—not their order in a reaction.

(Text continues on page 182.)

Coagulation factors

Factor I
• Fibrinogen
• Converts to fibrin when blood clots

Factor II
• Prothrombin
• Inactive precursor to thrombin

Factor III
• Tissue thromboplastin
• Converts prothrombin to thrombin as blood starts to clot

Factor IV
• Consists of calcium ions
• Required throughout the entire clotting sequence

Factor V
• Labile factor (proaccelerin)
• Functions during the combined pathway phase of the coagulation system

Factor VII
• Also known as serum prothrombin conversion accelerator or stable factor (proconvertin)
• Activated by Factor III in the extrinsic system

Factor VIII
• Antihemophilic factor
• Required during the intrinsic phase of the coagulation system

Factor IX
• Plasma thromboplastin component
• Required in the intrinsic phase of the coagulation system

Factor X
• Stuart factor (Stuart-Prower factor)
• Required in the combined pathway of the coagulation system

Factor XI
• Plasma thromboplastin antecedent
• Required in the intrinsic system

Factor XII
• Hageman factor
• Required in the intrinsic system

Factor XIII
• Fibrin-stabilizing factor
• Required to stabilize fibrin strands in the combined pathway phase of the coagulation system

Blood groups

- Determined by the presence or absence of genetically determined *antigens* or *agglutinogens* (glycoproteins) on the surface of RBCs
- Most clinically significant blood antigens are A, B, and Rh

ABO groups

- Involves testing for the presence of A and B antigens on RBCs
- Considered the most important system for classifying blood
  - Type A blood has A antigen on its surface
  - Type B blood has B antigen
  - Type AB blood has both A and B antigens
  - Type O blood has neither A nor B antigen

Rh typing

- Determines whether the Rh antigen (*Rh factor*) is present or absent in the blood
- Classifies blood with the Rh antigen as Rh-positive; blood without the Rh antigen as Rh-negative
- Recognizes that anti-Rh antibodies can appear only in a person who has become sensitized to the Rh antigen
  - Anti-Rh antibodies can appear in the blood of an Rh-negative person after entry of Rh-positive RBCs in the bloodstream (such as from transfusion of Rh-positive blood)
  - An Rh-negative female who carries an Rh-positive fetus may also acquire anti-Rh antibodies

Blood type compatibility

Blood group	Antibodies present in plasma	Compatible RBCs	Compatible plasma
Recipient			
O	Anti-A and anti-B	O	O, A, B, AB
A	Anti-B	A, O	A, AB
B	Anti-A	B, O	B, AB
AB	Neither anti-A nor anti-B	AB, A, B, O	AB
Donor			
O	Anti-A and anti-B	O, A, B, AB	O
A	Anti-B	A, AB	A, O
B	Anti-A	B, AB	B, O
AB	Neither anti-A nor anti-B	AB	AB, A, B, O

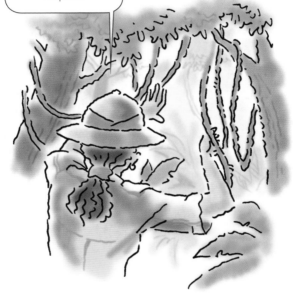

10

Immune system

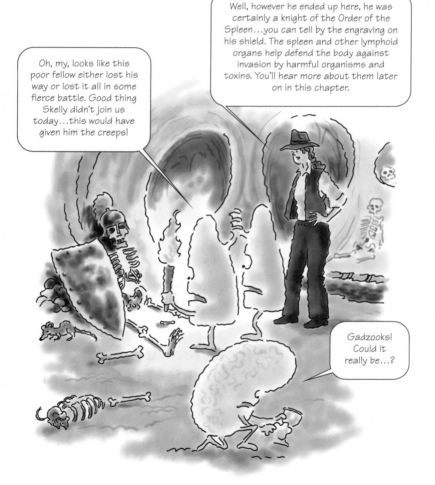

Immune system basics

- Defends the body against invasion by harmful organisms and chemical toxins
- Consists of organs and tissues referred to as "lymphoid" because they're involved with the growth, development, and dissemination of lymphocytes, one type of white blood cell (WBC)
- Has three major components: central lymphoid organs and tissue, peripheral lymphoid organs and tissue, and accessory lymphoid organs and tissue
- Closely related to the blood
  - Cells originate in bone marrow (as do blood cells)
  - Uses the bloodstream to transport its "troops" to the site of an invasion

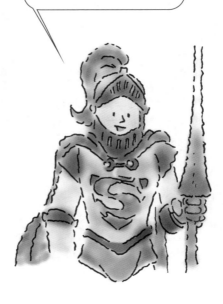

Immune system structures

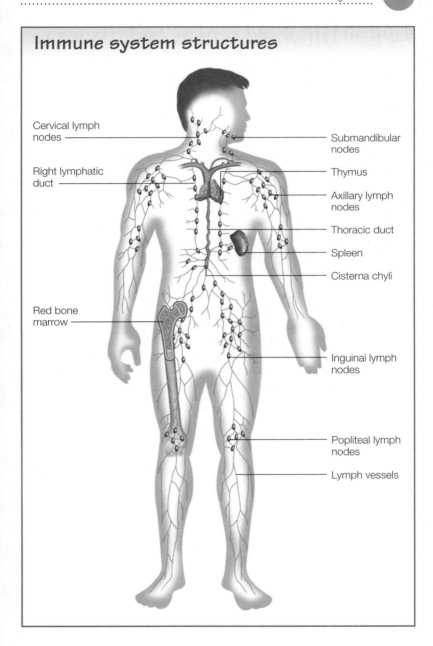

Cervical lymph nodes

Right lymphatic duct

Red bone marrow

Submandibular nodes

Thymus

Axillary lymph nodes

Thoracic duct

Spleen

Cisterna chyli

Inguinal lymph nodes

Popliteal lymph nodes

Lymph vessels

Central lymphoid organs and tissues

- Consists of bone marrow and the thymus
- Each plays a role in the development of B cells and T cells—the two major types of *lymphocytes*

Bone marrow

- Contains stem cells, which can develop into any of several different cell types
- Develops cells of the immune system and the blood from stem cells in a process called *hematopoiesis*
- Cells destined to become immune system cells develop into either *lymphocytes* or *phagocytes*
- Lymphocytes differentiate further to become either *B cells* or *T cells*
  - B cells and T cells are distributed throughout the lymphoid organs, especially the lymph nodes and spleen
  - Special receptors on them respond to specific antigen molecule shapes; in B cells, this receptor is called an *antibody*

Thymus

- A two-lobed mass of lymphoid tissue located over the base of the heart in the mediastinum in fetuses and infants
- Helps form T lymphocytes for several months after birth
- Gradually atrophies until only a remnant remains in adults
- "Trains" T cells to recognize other cells from the same body (self cells) and distinguish them from all other cells (nonself cells)

Stem cell differentiation

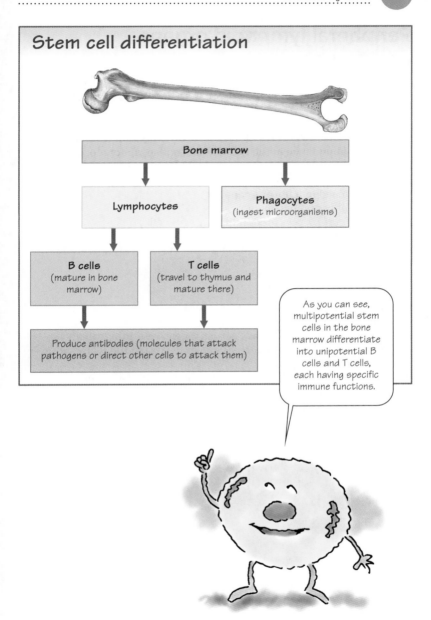

As you can see, multipotential stem cells in the bone marrow differentiate into unipotential B cells and T cells, each having specific immune functions.

Peripheral lymphoid organs and tissues

- Include the lymph nodes, the lymphatic vessels, and the spleen
- Work together to remove and destroy *antigens*

Lymph nodes

- Are small, oval structures along a network of lymph channels
- Found in abundance in the head, neck, axillae, abdomen, pelvis, and groin
- Help remove and destroy antigens in the blood and lymph
- Each enclosed in a fibrous capsule
- Contain three compartments:
  - *Superficial cortex* (predominantly of B cells)
  - *Deep cortex* and interfollicular areas (mostly T cells)
  - The *medulla* (numerous plasma cells that actively secrete *immunoglobulins*)

Lymph

- Contains a liquid portion as well as WBCs and antigens
- Collected from body tissues
- Seeps into *lymphatic vessels* across the vessels' thin walls
- Carried into the *subcapsular sinus* (or cavity) of the lymph nodes' *afferent lymphatic vessels*
- Flows through cortical sinuses and smaller radial medullary sinuses
- Carries antigens into the deep cortex and medullary sinuses, where phagocytic cells attack the antigens
- Leaves the node after being cleansed through *efferent lymphatic vessels* at the *hilum*

(Text continues on page 192.)

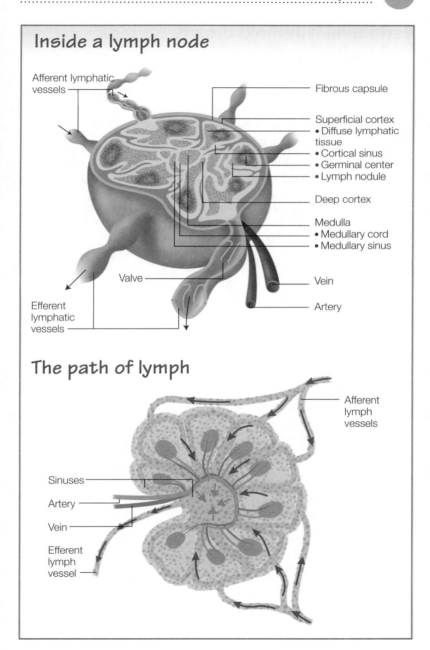

Inside a lymph node

Afferent lymphatic vessels

Fibrous capsule

Superficial cortex
• Diffuse lymphatic tissue
• Cortical sinus
• Germinal center
• Lymph nodule

Deep cortex

Medulla
• Medullary cord
• Medullary sinus

Valve

Vein

Artery

Efferent lymphatic vessels

The path of lymph

Afferent lymph vessels

Sinuses

Artery

Vein

Efferent lymph vessel

Peripheral lymphoid organs
and tissues *(continued)*
Lymph node regions
- Efferent lymphatic vessels drain into *lymph node chains*
- In turn, these empty into large lymph vessels, or trunks
- From there, lymph drains into the subclavian vein of the vascular system
- Numerous nodes line the lymphatic channels that drain a particular region, causing lymph to travel through more than one lymph node
  - For example, axillary nodes (located under the arm) filter drainage from the arms
  - Femoral nodes (in the inguinal region) filter drainage from the legs
- This arrangement prevents organisms that enter peripheral areas from migrating unchallenged to central areas

(Text continues on page 194.)

Lymph node chains and drainage

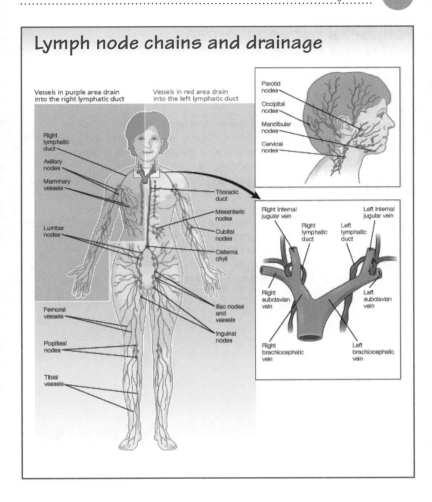

Vessels in purple area drain into the right lymphatic duct

Vessels in red area drain into the left lymphatic duct

Right lymphatic duct

Axillary nodes

Mammary vessels

Lumbar nodes

Femoral vessels

Popliteal nodes

Tibial vessels

Thoracic duct

Mesenteric nodes

Cubital nodes

Cisterna chyli

Iliac nodes and vessels

Inguinal nodes

Parotid nodes

Occipital nodes

Mandibular nodes

Cervical nodes

Right internal jugular vein

Right lymphatic duct

Left lymphatic duct

Left internal jugular vein

Right subclavian vein

Left subclavian vein

Right brachiocephalic vein

Left brachiocephalic vein

Peripheral lymphoid organs and tissues *(continued)*

Spleen

- Located in the left upper quadrant of the abdomen beneath the diaphragm
- Is a dark red, oval structure approximately the size of a fist
- Interior called *splenic pulp*, which contains white and red pulp
  - *White pulp*: surrounds branches of the splenic artery and contains compact masses of lymphocytes
  - *Red pulp*: consists of a network of blood-filled *sinusoids*; supported by a framework of reticular fibers and mononuclear phagocytes, along with some lymphocytes, plasma cells, and monocytes
- Contains phagocytes that engulf and break down worn-out RBCs and that also interact with lymphocytes to initiate an immune response
- Filters and removes bacteria and other foreign substances from the bloodstream
- Stores blood and 20% to 30% of platelets

Inside the spleen

Visceral surface

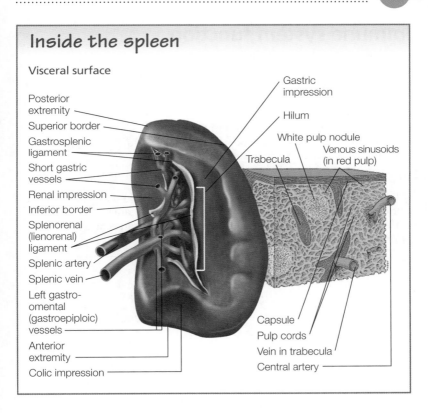

Posterior extremity

Superior border

Gastrosplenic ligament

Short gastric vessels

Renal impression

Inferior border

Splenorenal (lienorenal) ligament

Splenic artery

Splenic vein

Left gastro-omental (gastroepiploic) vessels

Anterior extremity

Colic impression

Gastric impression

Hilum

White pulp nodule

Venous sinusoids (in red pulp)

Trabecula

Capsule

Pulp cords

Vein in trabecula

Central artery

Immune system function

- Promotes *immunity* (the body's capacity to resist invading organisms and toxins, thereby preventing tissue and organ damage)
- Designed to recognize, respond to, and eliminate antigens, including bacteria, fungi, viruses, and parasites
- Preserves the body's internal environment by scavenging dead or damaged cells and patrolling for antigens
- Uses three basic strategies: protective surface phenomena, general host defenses, and specific immune responses

Protective surface phenomena

- Involves strategically placed physical, chemical, and mechanical barriers to prevent the entry of potentially harmful organisms
- Uses intact and healing skin and mucous membranes as a first line of defense

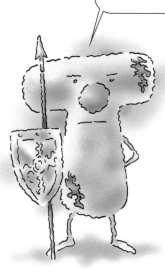

I'm part of the immune response team. Before things get that far, the body relies on intact and healing skin and mucous membranes, normal cell turnover, and a low pH to impede a bacterial invasion.

(Text continues on page 198.)

Protective surface phenomena

First line of defense

- Intact and healing skin and mucous membranes (prevent attachment of microorganisms)
- Normal cell turnover and low pH (further impede bacterial colonization)

Second line of defense

Organ system		Immune function
Nose		• Nasal hairs and turbulent airflow filter foreign materials. • Immunoglobulin in nasal secretions discourages microbe adherence.
Respiratory tract		• Mucous lining in the respiratory tract traps microorganisms. • Cilia lining the upper respiratory tract sweep dust particles and bacteria toward the mouth, preventing them from entering the lower respiratory tract.
GI tract		• Saliva, swallowing, peristalsis, and defecation mechanically remove bacteria. • Low pH of gastric secretions is bactericidal (bacteria-killing), rendering the stomach virtually free from live bacteria. • Resident bacteria in the rest of the GI system prevent other microorganisms from permanently making a home.
Urinary tract		• Urine flow, low urine pH, immunoglobulin and, in men, the bactericidal effects of prostatic fluid work together to impede bacterial colonization. • A series of sphincters inhibits bacterial migration.

Immune system function (continued)
General host defenses

- Involve nonspecific cellular responses to identify and remove an invader that has penetrated the skin or mucous membrane
- Trigger the *inflammatory response* as the first nonspecific response against an antigen
- Involve vascular and cellular changes, including the production and release of such chemical substances as heparin, histamine, and kinin
- Use polymorphonuclear leukocytes (*neutrophils, eosinophils, basophils,* and *mast cells*) in a big role in the inflammatory response

Neutrophils

- Increase dramatically in number in response to infection and inflammation
- Are the main constituent of pus and are highly mobile
- Engulf, digest, and dispose of invading organisms through a process called *phagocytosis*

Eosinophils

- Found in large numbers in the respiratory system and GI tract
- Multiply in allergic and parasitic disorders

Basophils and mast cells

- Have surface receptors for immunoglobulin (Ig) E
- Release mediators characteristic of the allergic response when their receptors are cross-linked by an IgE antigen complex

(Text continues on page 200.)

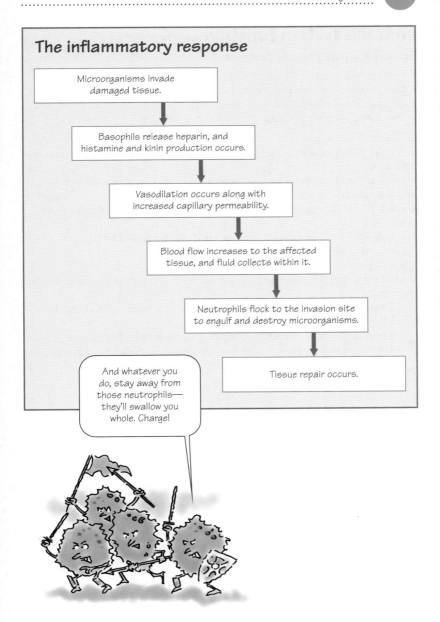

The inflammatory response

Microorganisms invade damaged tissue.

Basophils release heparin, and histamine and kinin production occurs.

Vasodilation occurs along with increased capillary permeability.

Blood flow increases to the affected tissue, and fluid collects within it.

Neutrophils flock to the invasion site to engulf and destroy microorganisms.

Tissue repair occurs.

And whatever you do, stay away from those neutrophils— they'll swallow you whole. Charge!

Immune system function *(continued)*

Specific immune responses

- Activated by particular microorganisms or molecules
- Can involve specialized sets of immune cells
- Classified as either *humoral immunity* or *cell-mediated immunity*
- Produced by lymphocytes (B cells and T cells)

Humoral immunity

- B cells divide and differentiate into plasma cells in response to an invading antigen
- Each plasma cell then produces and secretes large amounts of antigen-specific *immunoglobulins* into the bloodstream
- Each of the five types of immunoglobulins serves a particular function:
  - IgA, IgG, and IgM guard against viral and bacterial invasion
  - IgD acts as an antigen receptor of B cells
  - IgE causes an allergic response
- Immunoglobulins can work in one of several ways (depending on the antigen):
  - They can disable certain bacteria by linking with toxins that the bacteria produce
  - They can *opsonize* bacteria, making them targets for phagocytosis
  - Most commonly, they can link to antigens, causing the immune system to produce and circulate enzymes called *complement*

(Text continues on page 202.)

How macrophages accomplish phagocytosis

1 Chemotaxis

Chemotactic factors attract macrophages to the antigen site.

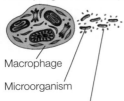

Macrophage

Microorganism

Chemotactic factors

2 Opsonization

Antibody (immunoglobulin G) or complement fragment coats the microorganism, enhancing macrophage binding to the antigen, now called an *opsinogen*.

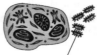

Opsonized microorganism

3 Ingestion

The macrophage extends its membrane around the opsonized microorganism, engulfing it within a vacuole *(phagosome)*.

Developing phagosome

4 Digestion

As the phagosome shifts away from the cell periphery, it merges with lysosomes, forming a *phagolysosome*, where antigen destruction occurs.

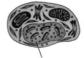

Phagolysosome

5 Chemotaxis

When digestion is complete, the macrophage expels digestive debris, including lysosomes, prostaglandins, complement components, and interferon, which continue to mediate the immune response.

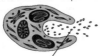

Digestive debris

Immune system function *(continued)*
Specific immune responses *(continued)*

Complement system

● Activated by a tissue injury or antigen–antibody reaction
● Bridges humoral and cell-mediated immunity and attracts phagocytic neutrophils and macrophages to the antigen site
● Consists of about 25 enzymes that "complement" the work of antibodies by aiding phagocytosis or destroying bacteria cells (through puncture of their cell membrane)

Cell-mediated immunity

● Protects the body against bacterial, viral, and fungal infections by inactivating the antigen
● Provides resistance against transplanted cells and tumor cells
● Causes T cells to move directly to attack invaders
● Involves three T-cell subgroups to trigger the response to infection:
  – *Helper T cells*: spur B cells to manufacture antibodies
  – *Effector T cells*: kill antigens and produce lymphokines (proteins that induce the inflammatory response and mediate the delayed hypersensitivity reaction)
  – *Suppressor T cells*: regulate T and B types of immune response

Immune response to bacterial invasion

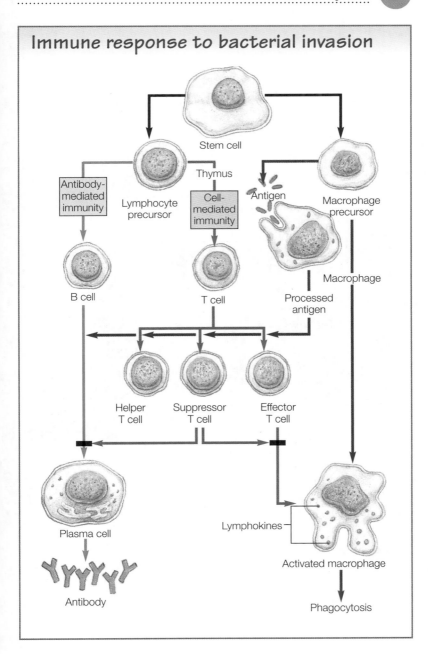

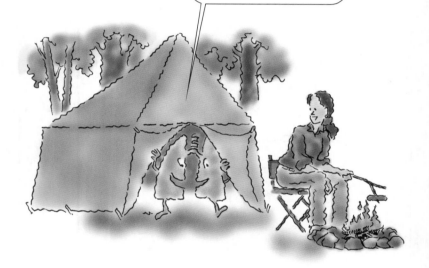

11

Respiratory system

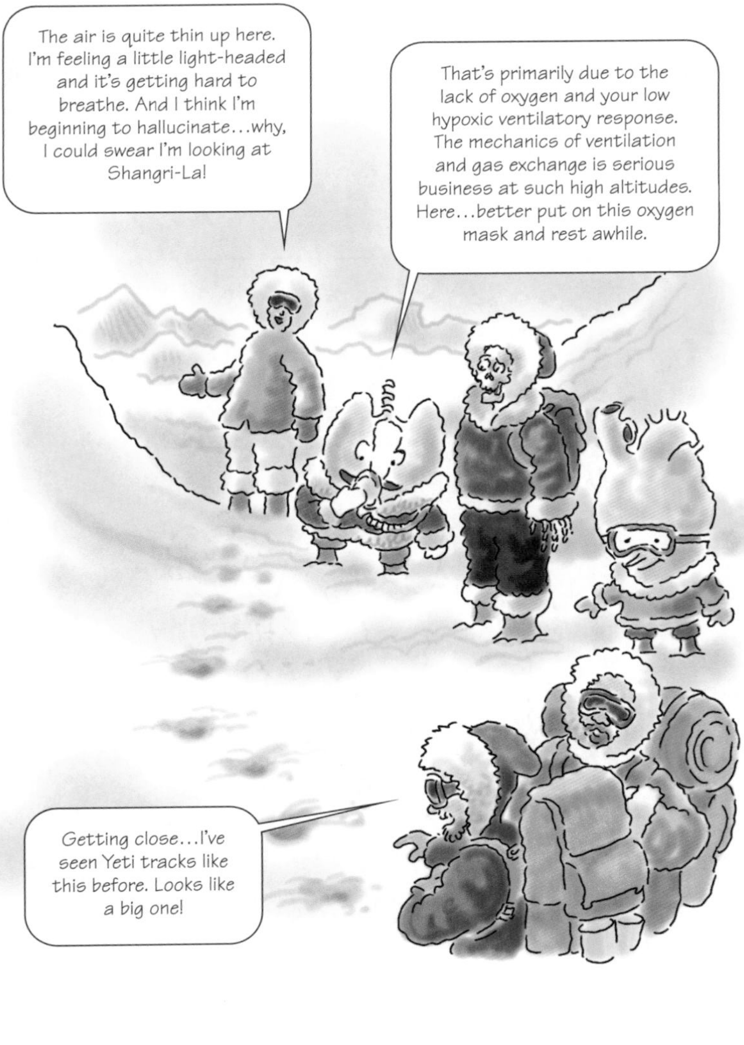

Respiratory system basics

- Maintains the exchange of oxygen and carbon dioxide in the lungs and tissues
- Helps regulate the body's acid-base balance
- Is composed of a *conducting zone* and a *respiratory zone*
  - The conducting zone consists of the continuous passageway that transports air in and out of the lungs (nose, pharynx, larynx, trachea, bronchi, and bronchioles)
  - The respiratory zone (composed of the bronchioles, alveolar ducts, and alveoli) performs gas exchange
- Consists of the upper respiratory tract, the lower respiratory tract, and the thoracic cavity

The respiratory system includes a cast of characters from the upper and lower respiratory tracts and the thoracic cavity, but I'm its star performer.

Structures of the respiratory system

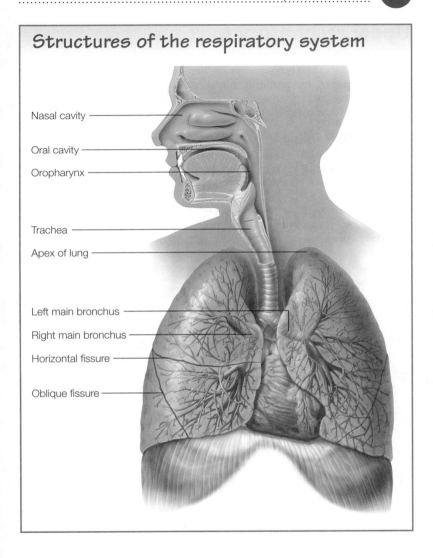

Nasal cavity

Oral cavity

Oropharynx

Trachea

Apex of lung

Left main bronchus

Right main bronchus

Horizontal fissure

Oblique fissure

Upper respiratory tract

● Consists primarily of the nose, mouth, nasopharynx, oropharynx, laryngopharynx, and larynx
● Filters, warms, and humidifies inspired air
● Responsible for detecting taste and smell and chewing and swallowing food

Nostrils and nasal passages

● Air enters the body through the nostrils (*nares*), where small hairs called *vibrissae* filter out dust and large foreign particles
● Air then passes into the two nasal passages, which are separated by the *septum*
● Cartilage forms the anterior walls of the nasal passages
● Bony structures (*conchae* or *turbinates*) form the posterior walls
  – The *conchae* warm and humidify air before it passes into the nasopharynx
  – Their mucus layer also traps finer foreign particles, which the *cilia* carry to the pharynx to be swallowed

Sinuses and nasopharynx

● Four pairs of paranasal sinuses open into the internal nose
● Sinuses provide speech resonance and produce mucus

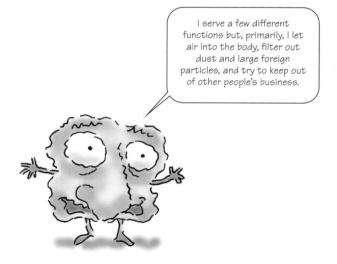

I serve a few different functions but, primarily, I let air into the body, filter out dust and large foreign particles, and try to keep out of other people's business.

(Text continues on page 210.)

Nasopharynx

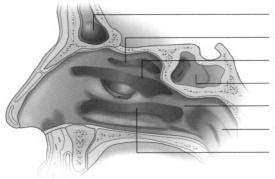

- Frontal sinus
- Nasal concha
- Middle nasal concha
- Sphenoid sinus
- Internal naris
- Nasopharynx
- Inferior nasal concha

Sinuses

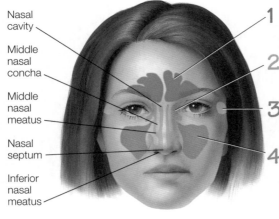

Nasal cavity

Middle nasal concha

Middle nasal meatus

Nasal septum

Inferior nasal meatus

1 Frontal sinuses, located above the eyebrows

2 Ethmoidal sinus, located behind the eyes and nose

3 Sphenoidal sinus, located behind the eyes

4 Maxillary sinus, located on the cheeks below the eyes

Upper respiratory tract *(continued)*
Oropharynx and laryngopharynx

- Oropharynx is the posterior wall of the mouth
- It connects the nasopharynx and the laryngopharynx
- The laryngopharynx extends to the esophagus and larynx

Larynx

- Larynx contains the vocal cords and connects the pharynx with the trachea
- It serves as the transition point between the upper and lower airways
- Muscles and cartilage form the walls of the larynx, including the large, shield-shaped thyroid cartilage situated just under the jawline
- The *epiglottis*, a flap of tissue that closes over the top of the larynx when the patient swallows, protects the patient from aspirating food or fluid into the lower airways

Oropharynx and laryngopharynx

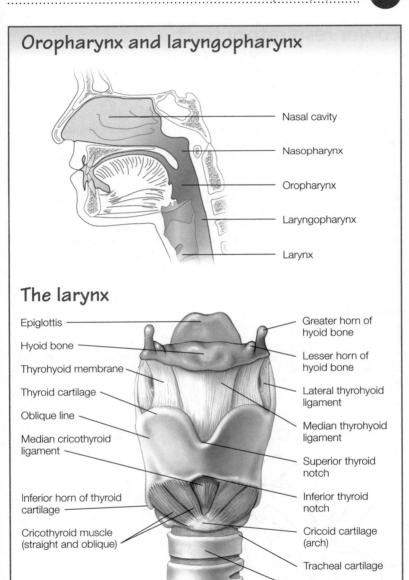

- Nasal cavity
- Nasopharynx
- Oropharynx
- Laryngopharynx
- Larynx

The larynx

Epiglottis

Hyoid bone

Thyrohyoid membrane

Thyroid cartilage

Oblique line

Median cricothyroid ligament

Inferior horn of thyroid cartilage

Cricothyroid muscle (straight and oblique)

Greater horn of hyoid bone

Lesser horn of hyoid bone

Lateral thyrohyoid ligament

Median thyrohyoid ligament

Superior thyroid notch

Inferior thyroid notch

Cricoid cartilage (arch)

Tracheal cartilage

Trachea

Lower respiratory tract

- Consists of the trachea, bronchi, and lungs
- Functionally divided into the *conducting airways* and the *acinus* (where gas exchange occurs)

Trachea

- Extends from the *cricoid cartilage* at the top to the carina (also called the *tracheal bifurcation*)
- C-shaped cartilage rings protect the trachea from collapsing

Bronchi

- The right mainstem bronchus—shorter, wider, and more vertical than the left—supplies air to the right lung
- The left mainstem bronchus delivers air to the left lung
- The mainstem bronchi divide into five lobar (secondary) bronchi
- Each lobar bronchus enters a lobe in each lung
- Each of the lobar bronchi branches into segmental bronchi (tertiary bronchi)
- The segments continue to branch into smaller bronchi, finally branching into bronchioles
- The larger bronchi consist of cartilage, smooth muscle, and epithelium
- As the bronchi become smaller, they lose cartilage and then smooth muscle; the smallest bronchioles consist of just a single layer of epithelial cells

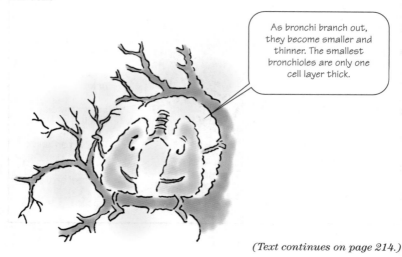

As bronchi branch out, they become smaller and thinner. The smallest bronchioles are only one cell layer thick.

(Text continues on page 214.)

Lower airways

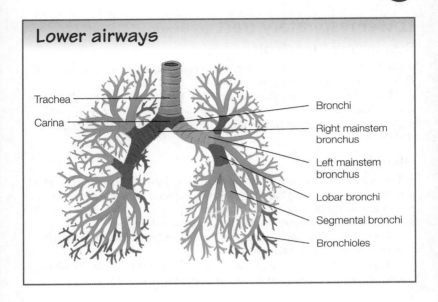

Trachea

Carina

Bronchi

Right mainstem bronchus

Left mainstem bronchus

Lobar bronchi

Segmental bronchi

Bronchioles

Lower respiratory tract (continued)

Respiratory bronchioles

- Each bronchiole includes terminal bronchioles and the acinus—the chief respiratory unit for gas exchange
- Within the acinus, terminal bronchioles branch into yet smaller respiratory bronchioles
- The respiratory bronchioles feed directly into alveoli at sites along their walls

Alveoli

- The respiratory bronchioles eventually become alveolar ducts, which terminate in clusters of capillary-swathed alveoli called *alveolar sacs*
- Gas exchange occurs through the alveoli
- Alveolar walls contain two basic epithelial cell types:
    - *Type I cells* (the most abundant) are thin, flat, squamous cells across which gas exchange occurs
    - *Type II cells* secrete *surfactant*, a substance that coats the alveolus and promotes gas exchange by lowering surface tension

(Text continues on page 216.)

Bronchioles

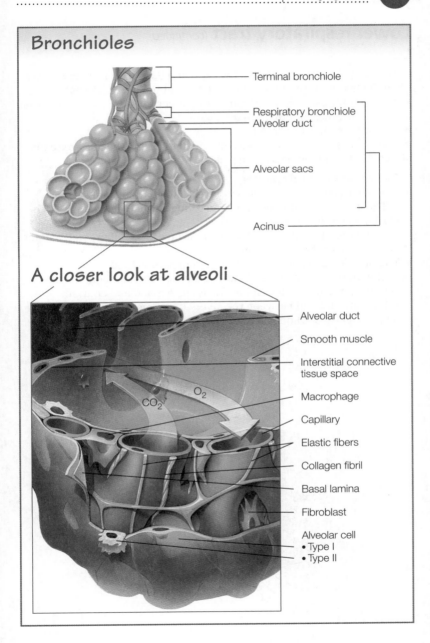

- Terminal bronchiole
- Respiratory bronchiole
- Alveolar duct
- Alveolar sacs
- Acinus

A closer look at alveoli

- Alveolar duct
- Smooth muscle
- Interstitial connective tissue space
- Macrophage
- Capillary
- Elastic fibers
- Collagen fibril
- Basal lamina
- Fibroblast
- Alveolar cell
  - Type I
  - Type II

CO_2 O_2

Lower respiratory tract *(continued)*

Lungs

- The lungs hang suspended in the right and left pleural cavities, straddling the heart, and anchored by root and pulmonary ligaments
- The right lung is shorter, broader, and larger than the left; it has three lobes and handles 55% of gas exchange
- The left lung has two lobes
- Each lung's concave base rests on the diaphragm; the apex extends about $\frac{1}{2}''$ (1.5 cm) above the first rib

Pleura and pleural cavities

- The pleura consists of a visceral layer and a parietal layer
  - The visceral pleura hugs the entire lung surface, including the areas between the lobes
  - The parietal pleura lines the inner surface of the chest wall and upper surface of the diaphragm
- The pleural cavity contains a thin film of serous fluid
  - The fluid lubricates the pleural surfaces, allowing them to slide smoothly against each other as the lungs expand and contract
  - It creates a bond between the layers that causes the lungs to move with the chest wall during breathing

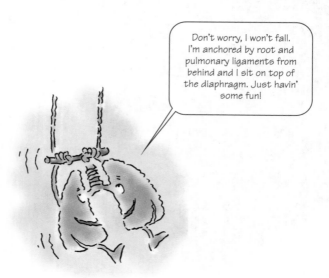

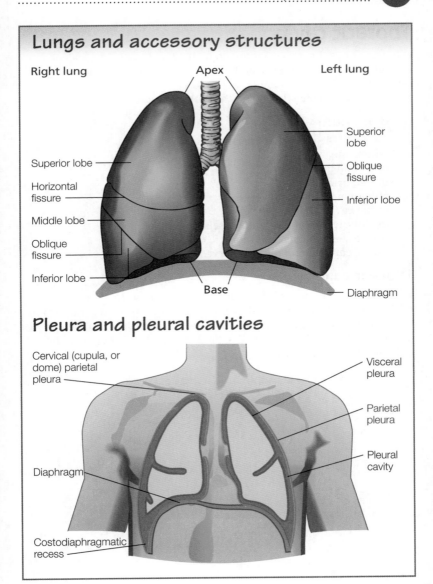

Lungs and accessory structures

Right lung
Apex
Left lung

Superior lobe

Oblique fissure

Inferior lobe

Superior lobe

Horizontal fissure

Middle lobe

Oblique fissure

Inferior lobe

Base

Diaphragm

Pleura and pleural cavities

Cervical (cupula, or dome) parietal pleura

Visceral pleura

Parietal pleura

Pleural cavity

Diaphragm

Costodiaphragmatic recess

Thoracic cavity

- Incorporates the area surrounded by the diaphragm, the scalene muscles and fasciae of the neck, and the ribs, intercostal muscles, vertebrae, sternum, and ligaments
- Includes the mediastinum and the thoracic cage

Mediastinum

- Consists of the space between the lungs
- Contains the:
  - heart and pericardium
  - thoracic aorta
  - pulmonary artery and veins
  - venae cavae and azygos veins
  - thymus, lymph nodes, and vessels
  - trachea, esophagus, and thoracic duct
  - vagus, cardiac, and phrenic nerves

Thoracic cage

- Composed of bone and cartilage; supports and protects the lungs
- The vertebral column and 12 pairs of ribs form the posterior portion
- The manubrium, sternum, xiphoid process, and ribs form the anterior portion, which protects the mediastinal organs that lie between the right and left pleural cavities

The thoracic cage

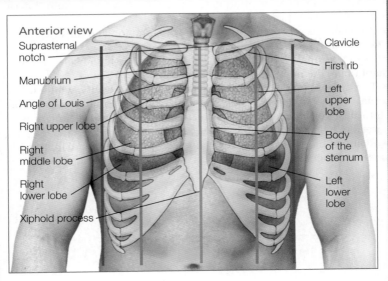

Anterior view
- Suprasternal notch
- Manubrium
- Angle of Louis
- Right upper lobe
- Right middle lobe
- Right lower lobe
- Xiphoid process
- Clavicle
- First rib
- Left upper lobe
- Body of the sternum
- Left lower lobe

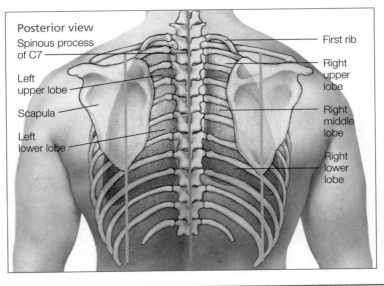

Posterior view
- Spinous process of C7
- Left upper lobe
- Scapula
- Left lower lobe
- First rib
- Right upper lobe
- Right middle lobe
- Right lower lobe

Inspiration and expiration

● Breathing involves inspiration (an active process) and expiration (a relatively passive process)
● Both actions rely on respiratory muscle function and the effects of pressure differences in the lungs
● During normal respiration, the external intercostal muscles aid the diaphragm, the major muscle of respiration
● The diaphragm descends to lengthen the chest cavity, while the external intercostal muscles contract to expand the anteroposterior diameter; this coordinated action causes a reduction in intrapleural pressure, and inspiration occurs
● Rising of the diaphragm and relaxation of the intercostal muscles causes an increase in intrapleural pressure, and expiration results

The diaphragm may be the major muscle of respiration, but we play a big part in respiration, too.

(Text continues on page 222.)

Inspiration and expiration

Inspiration

During inspiration, the diaphragm contracts (pressing the abdominal organs downward and forward) and the external intercostal muscles also contract. The rib cage expands, the volume of the thoracic cavity increases, and air rushes in to equalize the pressure.

Expiration

During expiration, the lungs passively recoil as the diaphragm and intercostal muscles relax, pushing air out of the lungs.

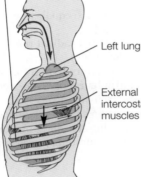

Left lung

External intercostal muscles

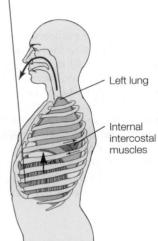

Left lung

Internal intercostal muscles

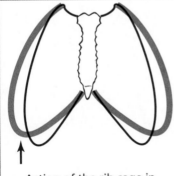

Action of the rib cage in inspiration

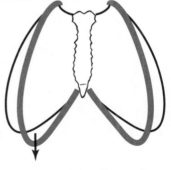

Action of the rib cage in expiration

Inspiration and expiration *(continued)*
Internal and external respiration
- Internal respiration (gas exchange in the tissues) occurs only through diffusion
- External respiration (gas exchange in the lungs) occurs through ventilation, pulmonary perfusion, and diffusion

Ventilation
- Involves the movement of gases in and out of the airways
- Results from differences in atmospheric and intrapulmonary pressures
- Consists of the following processes:
  - Before inspiration, intrapulmonary pressure equals atmospheric pressure (see #1 in the illustration at right)
  - The intrapulmonary atmospheric pressure gradient pulls air into the lungs until the two pressures are equal (#2)
  - During inspiration, the diaphragm and external intercostals muscles contract, enlarging the thorax; intrapleural pressure decreases and the lungs expand to fill the thoracic cavity (#3)
  - During normal expiration, the diaphragm slowly relaxes and the lungs and thorax passively return to resting size and position (#4)
  - During deep or forced expiration, intrapulmonary pressure rises above atmospheric pressure

(Text continues on page 224.)

Mechanics of ventilation

1

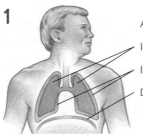

Atmospheric pressure (760 mm Hg)

Intrapulmonary pressure (760 mm Hg)

Intrapleural pressure (756 mm Hg)

Diaphragm

2

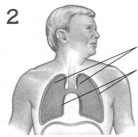

Atmospheric pressure (760 mm Hg)

Intrapulmonary pressure (760 mm Hg)

Intrapleural pressure (756 mm Hg)

3

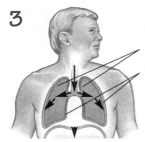

Atmospheric pressure (760 mm Hg)

Intrapulmonary pressure (758 mm Hg)

Intrapleural pressure (754 mm Hg)

4

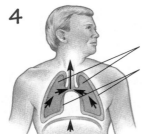

Atmospheric pressure (760 mm Hg)

Intrapulmonary pressure (763 mm Hg)

Intrapleural pressure (759 mm Hg)

Inspiration and expiration *(continued)*
Internal and external respiration *(continued)*

Pulmonary perfusion

● Refers to blood flow from the right side of the heart, through the pulmonary circulation, and into the left side of the heart; perfusion aids external respiration
● Normal pulmonary blood flow allows alveolar gas exchange
● Factors that may interfere with gas transport to the alveoli include:
– cardiac output less than the average of 5 L/minute
– elevations in pulmonary and systemic resistance
– abnormal or insufficient hemoglobin

Ventilation-perfusion mismatch

● *Shunting* (reduced ventilation) causes unoxygenated blood to move from the right side of the heart to the left side of the heart and into systemic circulation; it may result from physical defects or airway obstruction
● *Dead-space ventilation* (reduced perfusion) occurs when alveoli don't have adequate blood supply for gas exchange to occur, such as with pulmonary emboli and pulmonary infarction
● A *silent unit* (a combination of shunting and dead-space ventilation) occurs when little or no ventilation and perfusion are present, such as in cases of pneumothorax and acute respiratory distress syndrome

(Text continues on page 226.)

What happens in ventilation-perfusion mismatch

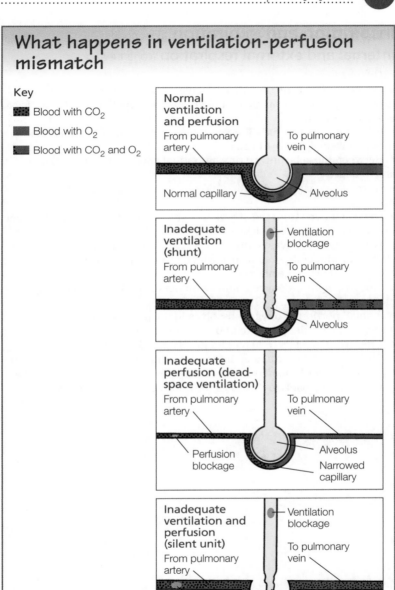

Key

- Blood with CO_2
- Blood with O_2
- Blood with CO_2 and O_2

Normal ventilation and perfusion
From pulmonary artery
To pulmonary vein
Normal capillary
Alveolus

Inadequate ventilation (shunt)
Ventilation blockage
From pulmonary artery
To pulmonary vein
Alveolus

Inadequate perfusion (dead-space ventilation)
From pulmonary artery
To pulmonary vein
Perfusion blockage
Alveolus
Narrowed capillary

Inadequate ventilation and perfusion (silent unit)
Ventilation blockage
From pulmonary artery
To pulmonary vein
Perfusion blockage
Alveolus

Inspiration and expiration *(continued)*

Internal and external respiration *(continued)*

Diffusion

● Oxygen and carbon dioxide molecules move between the alveoli and capillaries, always from an area of greater concentration to one of lesser concentration

● Both the alveolar epithelium and the capillary endothelium are composed of a single layer of cells

● Between these layers are tiny interstitial spaces filled with elastin and collagen

● Normally, oxygen and carbon dioxide move easily through these layers

● Oxygen moves from the alveoli into the bloodstream, where it's taken up by hemoglobin in the RBCs

● When oxygen arrives in the bloodstream, it displaces carbon dioxide (the by-product of metabolism), which diffuses from RBCs into the blood and then to the alveoli

● Most transported oxygen binds with hemoglobin to form oxyhemoglobin

● A small portion of oxygen dissolves in the plasma and can be measured as the partial pressure of oxygen in arterial blood, or Pao_2

● After oxygen binds to hemoglobin, RBCs travel to the tissues

● Through cellular diffusion, internal respiration occurs when RBCs release oxygen and absorb carbon dioxide; the RBCs then transport the carbon dioxide back to the lungs for removal during expiration

Gas exchange in an alveolus

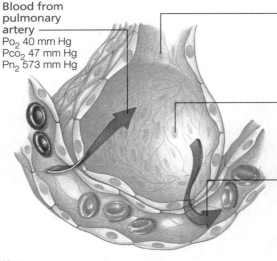

Blood from pulmonary artery
Po_2 40 mm Hg
Pco_2 47 mm Hg
Pn_2 573 mm Hg

Air entering lungs
Po_2 158 mm Hg
Pco_2 0.3 mm Hg
Pn_2 596 mm Hg
Ph_2o 5.7 mm Hg

Alveolar air
Po_2 100 mm Hg
Pco_2 40 mm Hg
Pn_2 573 mm Hg
Ph_2o 47 mm Hg

Blood to pulmonary vein
Po_2 97 mm Hg
Pco_2 40 mm Hg

Key
Po_2: partial pressure of oxygen
Pco_2: partial pressure of carbon dioxide
Pn_2: partial pressure of nitrogen
Ph_2o: partial pressure of water vapor

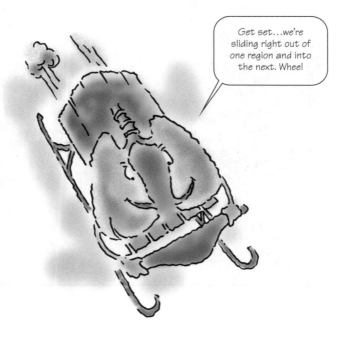

12

Gastrointestinal system

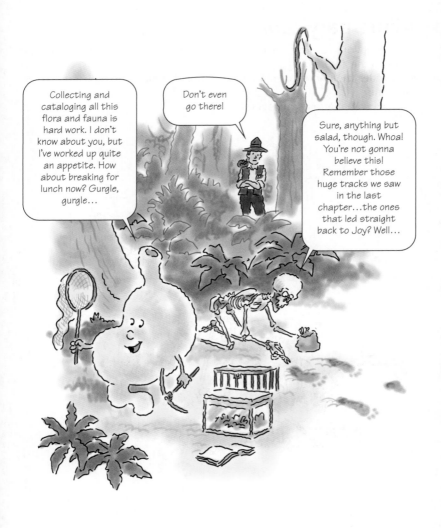

Gastrointestinal system basics

- Has two major components: the *alimentary canal* (also called the *GI tract*) and the *accessory GI organs*
- Serves two major functions:
  - *digestion,* or the breaking down of food and fluid into simple chemicals that can be absorbed into the bloodstream and transported throughout the body
  - *elimination* of waste products through excretion of stool

Alimentary canal

- Consists of a hollow muscular tube that begins in the mouth and extends to the anus
- Includes the pharynx, esophagus, stomach, small intestine, and large intestine
- Has a wall made up of several layers

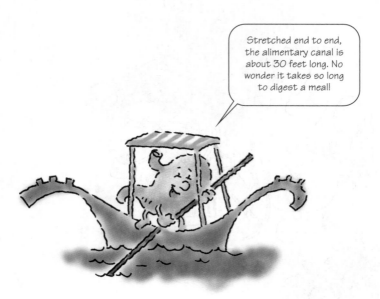

Stretched end to end, the alimentary canal is about 30 feet long. No wonder it takes so long to digest a meal!

(Text continues on page 232.)

Structures of the GI system

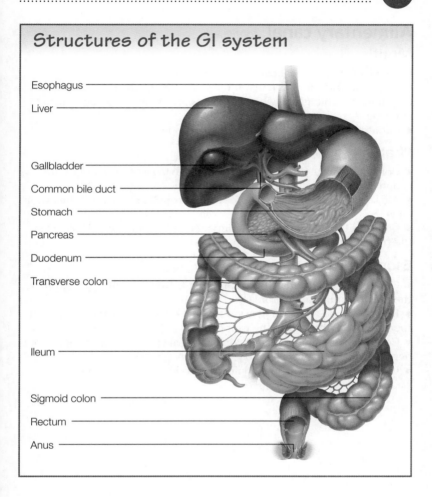

Esophagus

Liver

Gallbladder

Common bile duct

Stomach

Pancreas

Duodenum

Transverse colon

Ileum

Sigmoid colon

Rectum

Anus

Alimentary canal *(continued)*

Mouth

- Also called the buccal cavity or oral cavity
- Connects with the three major pairs of salivary glands (parotid, submandibular, sublingual), which secrete saliva to moisten food during chewing
- Initiates the mechanical breakdown of food

Pharynx

- Consists of a cavity that extends from the base of the skull to the esophagus
- Aids swallowing by grasping food and propelling it toward the esophagus
- Contains the *epiglottis*, a flap of connective tissue that closes over the trachea to prevent aspiration of food

Esophagus

- Consists of a muscular tube that extends from the pharynx through the mediastinum to the stomach
- Receives food from the pharynx; swallowing triggers the passage of food from the pharynx to the esophagus
- Contains a sphincter (the cricopharyngeal sphincter) at its upper border that must relax for food to enter the esophagus
- Uses peristalsis to propel liquids and solids into the stomach

(Text continues on page 234.)

Structures of the oral cavity

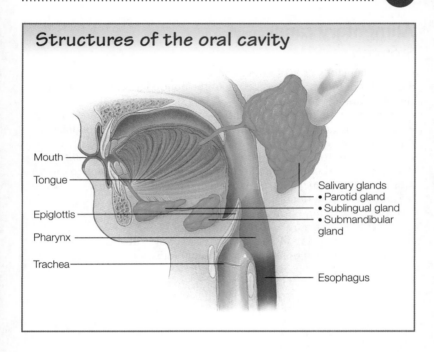

Mouth

Tongue

Epiglottis

Pharynx

Trachea

Salivary glands
• Parotid gland
• Sublingual gland
• Submandibular gland

Esophagus

Alimentary canal (continued)

Stomach

- Is a collapsible, pouchlike structure
- Resides in the left upper portion of the abdominal cavity, just below the diaphragm
- Attaches to the lower end of the esophagus at its upper border
- Has a lateral surface called the *greater curvature* and a medial surface, the *lesser curvature*
- Divided into four main regions: *cardia, fundus, body,* and *pylorus*
- Contains two sphincters: the *cardia* protects the entrance to the stomach and the *pyloric* guards the exit to the duodenum
- Has several functions, including:
  - serving as a temporary storage area for food
  - beginning digestion
  - breaking down food into *chyme,* a semifluid substance
  - moving gastric contents into the small intestine

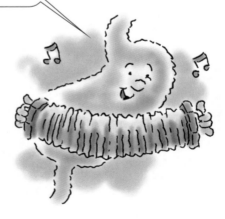

Because I'm a temporary storage tank for food, I can expand and contract to accommodate the amount consumed. Now that's what I call a squeezebox!

(Text continues on page 236.)

Stomach

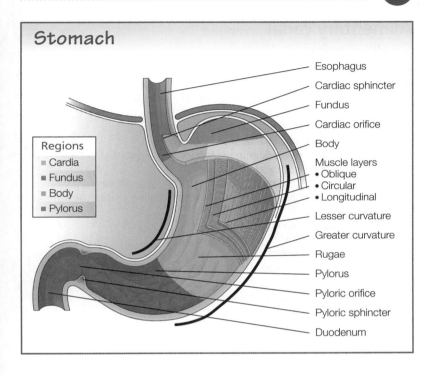

Regions
- Cardia
- Fundus
- Body
- Pylorus

Esophagus
Cardiac sphincter
Fundus
Cardiac orifice
Body
Muscle layers
• Oblique
• Circular
• Longitudinal
Lesser curvature
Greater curvature
Rugae
Pylorus
Pyloric orifice
Pyloric sphincter
Duodenum

Alimentary canal *(continued)*
Small intestine

- Is the longest organ of the GI tract
- Has three major divisions: the *duodenum, jejunum,* and *ileum*
- Contains structural features on its intestinal wall that increase its absorptive surface area:
    - *Plicae* circulares: circular folds of the mucosa
    - *Villi*: fingerlike projections on the mucosa
    - *Microvilli*: tiny cytoplasmic projections on epithelial cells
- Contains other structures:
    - *Intestinal crypts*: simple glands in the grooves separating villi
    - *Peyer's patches*: collections of lymphatic tissue within the submucosa
    - *Brunner's glands*: secrete mucus
- Has four main functions:
    - Completes food digestion
    - Absorbs food molecules through its wall into the circulatory system, which then delivers them to body cells
    - Secretes hormones that help control the secretion of bile, pancreatic fluid, and intestinal fluid

(Text continues on page 238.)

Small intestine

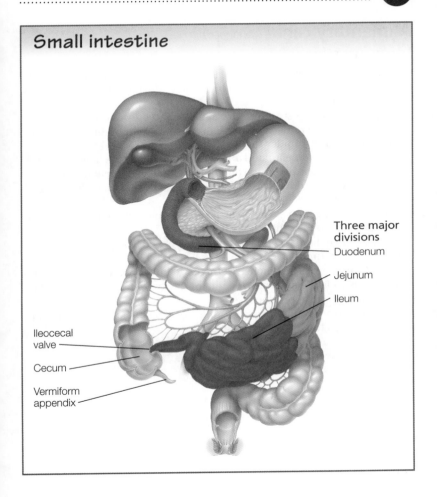

Three major divisions
Duodenum

Jejunum

Ileum

Ileocecal valve

Cecum

Vermiform appendix

Alimentary canal *(continued)*

Large intestine

- Extends from the ileocecal valve (the valve between the ileum of the small intestine and the first segment of the large intestine) to the anus
- Has six segments:
  - *Cecum*: a saclike structure that makes up the first few inches
  - *Ascending colon*: rises on the right posterior abdominal wall, and then turns sharply under the liver at the hepatic flexure
  - *Transverse colon*: situated above the small intestine, passes horizontally across the abdomen and below the liver, stomach, and spleen, and turns downward at the left colic flexure (also known as the *splenic flexure*)
  - *Descending colon*: starts near the spleen and extends down the left side of the abdomen into the pelvic cavity
  - *Sigmoid colon*: descends through the pelvic cavity, where it becomes the rectum
  - *Rectum*: the last few inches of the large intestine; terminates at the *anus*, which is the external opening of the large intestine that allows expulsion of waste products
- Performs several functions, including absorbing water, secreting mucus, and eliminating digestive wastes

(Text continues on page 240.)

Large intestine

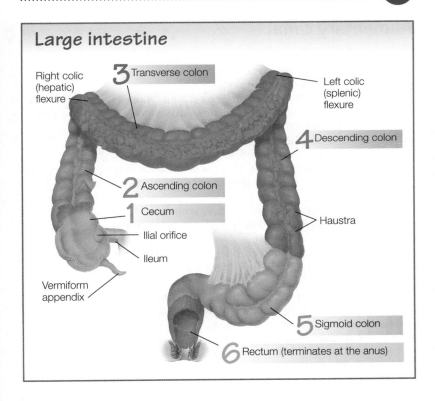

Right colic (hepatic) flexure

3 Transverse colon

Left colic (splenic) flexure

4 Descending colon

2 Ascending colon

1 Cecum

Ilial orifice

Ileum

Vermiform appendix

Haustra

5 Sigmoid colon

6 Rectum (terminates at the anus)

Alimentary canal *(continued)*
GI tract wall structures

- *Mucosa*: the innermost layer
  - Also called the *tunica mucosa*
  - Consists of epithelial and surface cells and loose connective tissue
  - Contains *villi*, fingerlike projections that secrete gastric and protective juices and absorb nutrients
- *Submucosa*: encircles the mucosa
  - Also called the *tunica submucosa*
  - Composed of loose connective tissue, blood and lymphatic vessels, and a nerve network called the *submucosal plexus*, or *Meissner's plexus*
- *Tunica muscularis*: lies around the submucosa
  - Composed of skeletal muscle in the mouth, pharynx, and upper esophagus
  - Made up of longitudinal and circular smooth muscle fibers elsewhere in the tract; aids in peristalsis and, at points, circular fibers thicken to form sphincters
  - In the large intestine, these fibers gather into three narrow bands (*taeniae coli*) down the middle of the colon and pucker the intestine into characteristic pouches (*haustra*)
- *Visceral peritoneum*: the GI tract's outer covering
  - Covers most of the abdominal organs
  - Lies next to an identical layer, the *parietal peritoneum*, which lines the abdominal cavity

GI tract wall structures

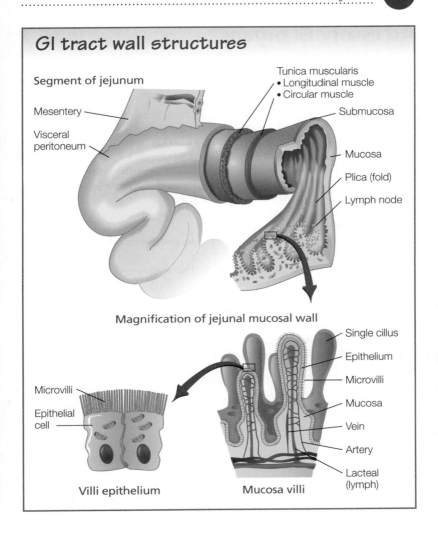

Segment of jejunum

- Mesentery
- Visceral peritoneum
- Tunica muscularis
  - Longitudinal muscle
  - Circular muscle
- Submucosa
- Mucosa
- Plica (fold)
- Lymph node

Magnification of jejunal mucosal wall

- Single cillus
- Epithelium
- Microvilli
- Mucosa
- Vein
- Artery
- Lacteal (lymph)

- Microvilli
- Epithelial cell

Villi epithelium   **Mucosa villi**

Accessory GI organs

- Contribute hormones, enzymes, and bile, which are vital to digestion
- Include the liver, gallbladder, and pancreas

Liver

- Enclosed in a fibrous capsule in the right upper quadrant of the abdomen
- Covered mostly by the *lesser omentum,* a fold of peritoneum, which also anchors it to the lesser curvature of the stomach
- Passing through the lesser omentum are the *hepatic artery,* the *hepatic portal vein,* the common bile duct, and the hepatic veins
- Contains *lobules,* the liver's functional units
  - Each consists of a plate of hepatic cells (*hepatocytes*) that encircle a central vein and radiate outward
  - Separating these plates are *sinusoids,* the liver's capillary system
- Serves many functions
  - Metabolizes carbohydrates, fats, and proteins
  - Detoxifies blood
  - Converts ammonia to urea for excretion
  - Synthesizes plasma proteins, nonessential amino acids, vitamins, and essential nutrients
  - Secretes *bile*—an alkaline, greenish liquid composed of water, cholesterol, bile salts, and phospholipids

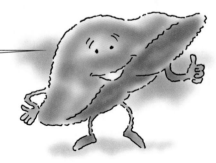

Not to brag, but I am the largest gland in the body and crucial to metabolic processes. Why, they couldn't get along without me!

(Text continues on page 244.)

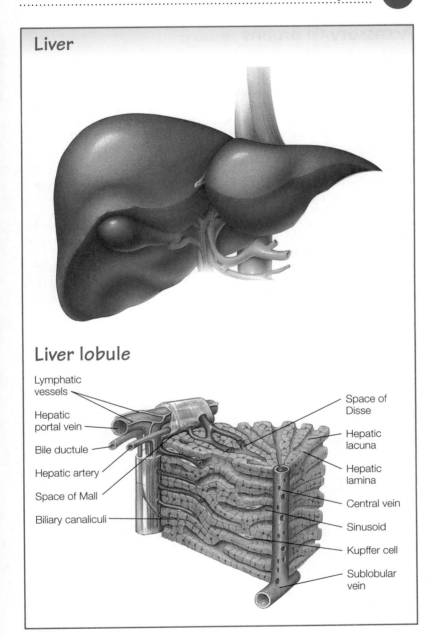

Liver

Liver lobule

- Lymphatic vessels
- Hepatic portal vein
- Bile ductule
- Hepatic artery
- Space of Mall
- Biliary canaliculi

- Space of Disse
- Hepatic lacuna
- Hepatic lamina
- Central vein
- Sinusoid
- Kupffer cell
- Sublobular vein

Accessory GI organs (continued)

Liver (continued)

Ducts

- Serve to transport bile through the GI tract
- Bile exits the liver through bile ducts (canaliculi) that merge into the right and left hepatic ducts to form the common hepatic duct
- The common hepatic duct joins the cystic duct from the gallbladder to form the common bile duct, which leads to the duodenum

Bile

- Works to *emulsify* (break down) fat and promote intestinal absorption of fatty acids, cholesterol, and other lipids
- Is continuously secreted by the liver
- Production may increase from stimulation of the vagus nerve, release of the hormone secretin, increased blood flow in the liver, and the presence of fat in the intestine
- By combining bile salts with bile pigments (biliverdin and bilirubin, the waste products of red blood cell breakdown) and cholesterol, the liver recycles about 80% of bile salts into bile

(Text continues on page 246.)

GI hormones: production and function

When stimulated, GI structures secrete five hormones. Each hormone plays a different role in digestion.

Hormone and production site	Stimulating factor or agent	Function
Gastrin Produced in pyloric antrum and duodenal mucosa	• Pyloric antrum distention • Vagal stimulation • Protein digestion products • Alcohol	Stimulates gastric secretion and motility
Gastric inhibitory peptides Produced in duodenal and jejunal mucosa	• Gastric acid • Fats • Fat digestion products	Inhibits gastric secretion and motility
Secretin Produced in duodenal and jejunal mucosa	• Gastric acid • Fat digestion products • Protein digestion products	Stimulates secretion of bile and alkaline pancreatic fluid
Cholecystokinin Produced in duodenal and jejunal mucosa	• Fat digestion products • Protein digestion products	Stimulates gallbladder contraction and secretion of enzyme-rich pancreatic fluid
Motilin Produced in duodenal mucosa	• Gastric acid • Fats	Increases gastric motility

Accessory GI organs *(continued)*

Gallbladder

- Pear-shaped organ joined to the ventral surface of the liver by the cystic duct
- Covered with visceral peritoneum
- Stores and concentrates bile produced by the liver
- Releases bile into the common bile duct (formed by the cystic duct and common hepatic duct) for delivery to the duodenum in response to the contraction and relaxation of the sphincter of Oddi

Pancreas

- A somewhat flat organ that lies behind the stomach
- Consists of a head, body, and tail
- Beta cells secrete *insulin* to promote carbohydrate metabolism (endocrine function)
- Alpha cells secrete *glucagon* to stimulate glycogenolysis in the liver (endocrine function)
- Produces enzymes that aid in digestion (exocrine function)

Gallbladder and pancreas

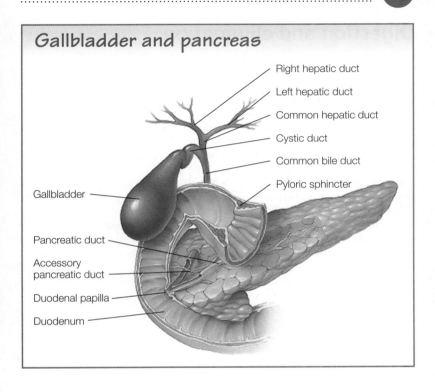

Right hepatic duct

Left hepatic duct

Common hepatic duct

Cystic duct

Common bile duct

Pyloric sphincter

Gallbladder

Pancreatic duct

Accessory pancreatic duct

Duodenal papilla

Duodenum

Digestion and elimination

- Digestion starts in the oral cavity, where chewing (*mastication*), salivation (the beginning of starch digestion), and swallowing (*deglutition*) take place
- Swallowing is initiated by a neural pattern
  - Food pushed to the back of the mouth stimulates swallowing receptor areas that surround the pharyngeal opening
  - These receptor areas transmit impulses to the brain by way of the sensory portions of the trigeminal and glossopharyngeal nerves
  - The brain's swallowing center (located in the brainstem) then relays motor impulses to the esophagus by way of the trigeminal, glossopharyngeal, vagus, and hypoglossal nerves, causing swallowing to occur
- When a person swallows, the hypopharyngeal sphincter in the upper esophagus relaxes, allowing food to enter the esophagus
- In the esophagus, the glossopharyngeal nerve activates peristalsis, which moves the food down toward the stomach
- Glands in the esophageal mucosal layer secrete mucus, which lubricates the bolus and protects the mucosal membrane from damage caused by poorly chewed foods

(Text continues on page 250.)

What happens in swallowing

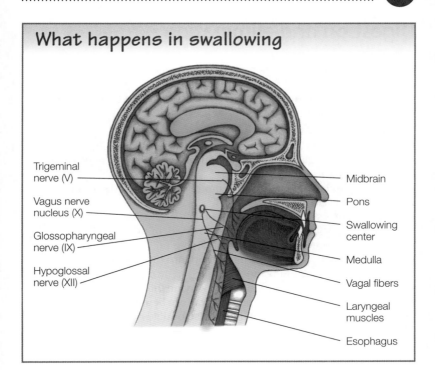

Digestion and elimination (continued)

Cephalic phase of digestion
● By the time the food bolus is traveling toward the stomach, the *cephalic phase* of digestion has already begun
● In this phase, the stomach secretes digestive juices (hydrochloric acid [HCl] and pepsin)

Gastric phase of digestion
● When food enters the stomach through the cardiac sphincter, the stomach wall stretches, stimulating the stomach to release *gastrin* (initiating the *gastric phase*)
● Gastrin stimulates the stomach's motor functions and secretion of gastric juice by the gastric glands
  – Gastric juices are highly acidic (pH of 0.9 to 1.5)
  – These digestive secretions consist mainly of pepsin, HCl, intrinsic factor, and proteolytic enzymes
● Peristaltic contractions churn the food into tiny particles and mix it with gastric juices, forming *chyme*
● Stronger peristaltic waves move the chyme into the antrum, where it backs up against the pyloric sphincter before being released into the duodenum, triggering the intestinal phase of digestion

(Text continues on page 252.)

Sites of gastric secretion

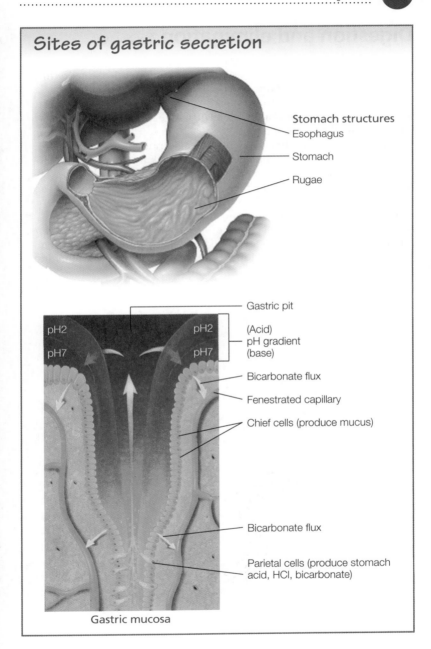

Stomach structures
Esophagus
Stomach
Rugae

Gastric pit

pH2 (Acid)
pH7 pH gradient (base)

Bicarbonate flux
Fenestrated capillary
Chief cells (produce mucus)

Bicarbonate flux

Parietal cells (produce stomach acid, HCl, bicarbonate)

Gastric mucosa

Digestion and elimination (continued)

Intestinal phase of digestion

- The *enterogastric reflex* causes the duodenum to release secretin and gastric-inhibiting peptide and the jejunum to secrete cholecystokinin—all of which act to decrease gastric motility
- Intestinal contractions and various digestive secretions break down carbohydrates, proteins, and fats
- These nutrients are then available for absorption into the bloodstream (along with water and electrolytes), making them available for use by the body
- Circular projections of the intestinal mucosa (*Kerckring's folds*) are covered by villi, increasing the surface area for absorption
- The large intestine continues the absorptive process
- *Escherichia coli, Enterobacter aerogenes, Clostridium perfringens,* and *Lactobacillus bifidus*—all found in the large intestine—help synthesize vitamin K and break down cellulose into a usable carbohydrate

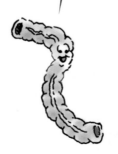

Some bacteria are normally present in the GI system. They help synthesize vitamin K and break down cellulose into a usable carbohydrate.

Inside the small intestine

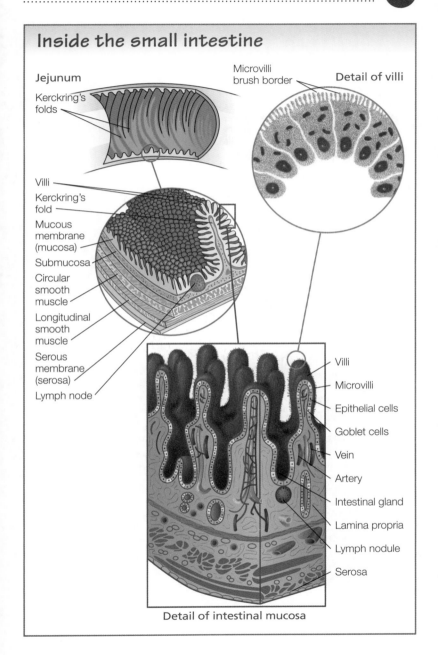

Jejunum

Kerckring's folds

Microvilli brush border

Detail of villi

Villi

Kerckring's fold

Mucous membrane (mucosa)

Submucosa

Circular smooth muscle

Longitudinal smooth muscle

Serous membrane (serosa)

Lymph node

Villi

Microvilli

Epithelial cells

Goblet cells

Vein

Artery

Intestinal gland

Lamina propria

Lymph nodule

Serosa

Detail of intestinal mucosa

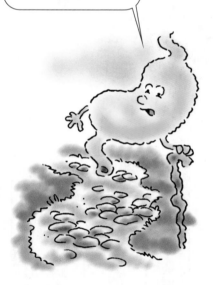

13

Nutrition and metabolism

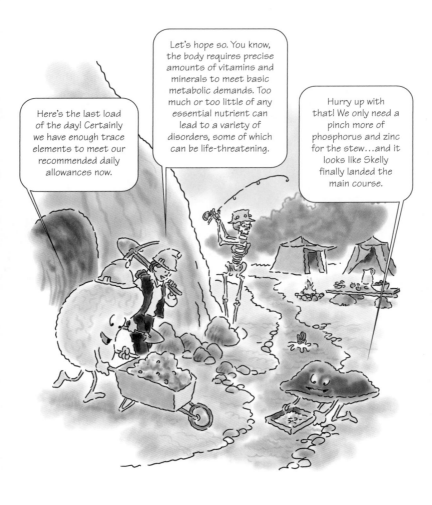

Components of nutrition

- *Nutrition*: the intake, assimilation, and utilization of nutrients
  - The crucial nutrients in foods must be broken down into components for use by the body
  - Within cells, the products of digestion undergo further chemical reactions
- *Metabolism*: the sum of the chemical reactions occurring within cells, when food substances are transformed into energy or materials that the body can use or store
- The body needs a continual supply of water and various nutrients for growth and repair
- The three major types of nutrients: carbohydrates, proteins, and lipids
- *Vitamins*: contribute to the enzyme reactions that promote the metabolism of carbohydrates, proteins, and lipids
- *Minerals*: participate in such essential functions as enzyme metabolism and membrane transfer of essential elements

(Text continues on page 258.)

Food group recommendations

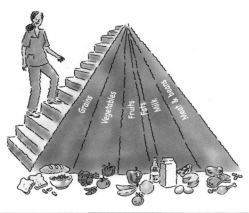

Grains	Vegetables	Fruits	Milk	Meats & beans
• Make one-half of your grains whole. • Eat at least 3 oz of whole-grain cereals, breads, crackers, rice, or pasta every day. • 1 oz is about 1 slice of bread, about 1 cup of breakfast cereal, or ½ cup of cooked rice, cereal, or pasta.	• Vary your veggies. • Eat more dark-green veggies like broccoli, spinach, and other dark leafy greens. • Eat more orange veggies, like carrots and sweet potatoes. • Eat more dry beans and peas like pinto beans, kidney beans, and lentils.	• Focus on fruits. • Eat a variety of fruit. • Choose fresh, frozen, canned, or dried fruit. • Go easy on fruit juices.	• Consume calcium-rich foods. • Go low-fat or fat-free when you choose milk, yogurt, and other milk products. • If you don't or can't consume milk, choose lactose-free products or other calcium sources, such as fortified foods and beverages.	• Go lean with protein. • Choose low-fat or lean meats and poultry. • Bake it, broil it, or grill it. • Vary your protein routine; choose more fish, beans, peas, nuts, and seeds.

For a 2,000 calorie diet, you need the amounts below from each food group. To find the amounts that are right for you, go to MyPyramid.gov.

Eat 6 oz every day.	Eat 2½ cups every day.	Eat 2 cups every day.	Get 3 cups every day; for kids ages 2 to 8, 2 cups.	Eat 5½ oz every day.

Components of nutrition (continued)

Carbohydrates

● Consist of organic compounds composed of carbon, hydrogen, and oxygen that convert to glucose in the body

● *Simple carbohydrates*: include the sugars in fruits, vegetables, dairy products, and foods made with processed sugar; they raise the blood glucose level quickly

● *Complex carbohydrates*: include the starches and fiber in breads, grains, and beans; they raise the blood glucose level more slowly

● Sugars are classified as *monosaccharides*, *disaccharides*, and *polysaccharides*

Proteins

● Are complex nitrogenous organic compounds containing amino acid chains; some also contain sulfur and phosphorus

● Used mainly for growth and repair of body tissues; when used for energy, they yield 4 kcal/g

● May combine with lipids to form *lipoproteins* or with carbohydrates to form *glycoproteins*

● Consist of building blocks called *amino acids*; each amino acid contains a carbon atom to which a carboxyl (COOH) group and an amino group are attached

(Text continues on page 260.)

Carbohydrates

Monosaccharides

- Are simple sugars
- Can't be broken down by the digestive process
- Are absorbed through the small intestine
- Examples: glucose (dextrose), fructose, galactose

Disaccharides

- Are synthesized from monosaccharides
- Consist of two monosaccharides minus a water molecule
- Examples: sucrose, lactose, maltose

Polysaccharides

- Are synthesized from monosaccharides
- Are ingested and broken down into simple sugars and used for fuel
- Consist of a long chain of monosaccharides linked by glycoside bonds
- Examples: glycogen, starch

Proteins

Protein is:

- required for normal growth and development
- broken down by the body as a source of energy when the supply of carbohydrates and fats is inadequate
- stored in muscle, bone, skin, cartilage, and lymph

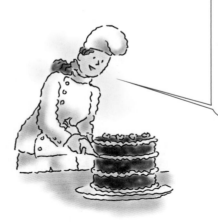

Carbohydrates are a quick source of energy when the body needs it; proteins can also be broken down and used for energy when the supply of carbs and fats is low. How about a slice of quick energy?

Components of nutrition *(continued)*

Lipids

● Are organic compounds that don't dissolve in water but do dissolve in alcohol and other organic solvents
● Yield about 9 kcal/g when used for energy
● Include fats, phospholipids, and sterols
● *Triglyceride*: a fat that contains three molecules of fatty acid combined with one molecule of glycerol
  – *Glycerol*: a three-carbon compound with an OH group attached to each carbon atom
  – The COOH group on each fatty acid molecule joins to one OH group on the glycerol molecule; this results in the release of a water molecule
● *Phospholipids*: complex lipids that are similar to fat but have a phosphorus- and nitrogen-containing compound that replaces one of the fatty acid molecules; are major structural components of cell membranes
● *Sterols*: complex molecules in which the carbon atoms form four cyclic structures attached to various side chains; examples include cholesterol, bile salts, and sex hormones

(Text continues on page 262.)

Fats

Triglycerides

- Account for about 95% of the fat in food
- Are the major storage form of fat in the body
- Contain fatty acids that can be saturated or unsaturated

Saturated fatty acid

- Saturated or filled with hydrogen ions
- Found in meat, poultry, full-fat dairy products, and tropical oils (such as palm and coconut oils)

Unsaturated fatty acid

- Not completely filled with hydrogen ions
- Usually soft or liquid at room temperature
- Originate from plant fat and oils
- Have lower melting points
- Can become rancid when exposed to extended periods of light and oxygen

Trans fats

- Produced by hydrogenation
- Found in vegetable shortening, certain margarines, crackers, cookies, snack foods, and other foods made with hydrogenated oils

Phospholipids

- Complex lipids that are similar to fat but that have a phosphorus- and nitrogen-containing compound that replaces one of the fatty acid molecules
- Are major structural components of cell membranes
- Occur naturally in all foods

Sterols

- Complex molecules in which the carbon atoms form four cyclic structures attached to various side chains
- Contain no glycerol or fatty acid molecules
- Example: cholesterol

Cholesterol

- Most common sterol
- Manufactured daily by the body
- Produced and filtered by the liver
- Necessary for the production of some hormones (estrogen, cortisone, epinephrine, and testosterone)

Components of nutrition *(continued)*

Vitamins

- Are organic compounds needed in small quantities for normal metabolism, growth, and development
- Classified as water-soluble or fat-soluble
- Water-soluble vitamins:
  - Aren't stored in the body
  - Must be replaced daily
  - Include the B complex and C vitamins
- Fat-soluble vitamins:
  - Must dissolve in fat before being absorbed by the bloodstream
  - Stored in the liver and body tissues when excess amounts exist (therefore, they don't need to be ingested daily)
  - Include vitamins A, D, E, and K

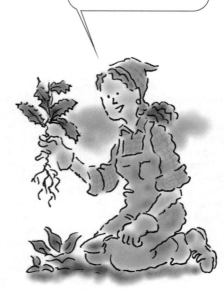

Nature provides a ready source of all the vitamins your body needs on a daily basis to stay healthy and strong. Can you dig it?

(Text continues on page 264.)

Guide to vitamins

Vitamin	Major functions
Water-soluble vitamins	
Vitamin C (ascorbic acid)	Collagen production, fine bone and tooth formation, iodine conservation, healing, red blood cell (RBC) formation, infection resistance
Vitamin B_1 (thiamine)	Blood formation, carbohydrate metabolism, circulation, digestion, growth, learning ability, muscle tone maintenance, central nervous system (CNS) maintenance
Vitamin B_2 (riboflavin)	RBC formation; energy metabolism; cell respiration; epithelial, eye, and mucosal tissue maintenance
Vitamin B_6 (pyridoxine)	Antibody formation, digestion, deoxyribonucleic acid (DNA) and ribonucleic acid (RNA) synthesis, fat and protein utilization, amino acid metabolism, hemoglobin production, CNS maintenance
Folic acid (folacin, pteroylglutamic acid)	Cell growth and reproduction, digestion, liver function, DNA and RNA formation, protein metabolism, RBC formation
Niacin (nicotinic acid, nicotinamide, niacinamide)	Circulation, cholesterol level reduction, growth, hydrochloric acid production, metabolism (carbohydrate, protein, fat), sex hormone production
Vitamin B_{12} (cyanocobalamin)	RBC formation, cellular and nutrient metabolism, tissue growth, nerve cell maintenance, appetite stimulation
Fat-soluble vitamins	
Vitamin A	Body tissue repair and maintenance, infection resistance, bone growth, nervous system development, cell membrane metabolism and structure, night vision
Vitamin D (calciferol)	Calcium and phosphorus metabolism (bone formation), myocardial function, nervous system maintenance, normal blood clotting
Vitamin E (tocopherol)	Aging retardation, anticlotting factor, diuresis, fertility, lung protection (antipollution), male potency, muscle and nerve cell membrane maintenance, myocardial perfusion, serum cholesterol reduction
Vitamin K (menadione)	Liver synthesis of prothrombin and other blood-clotting factors

Components of nutrition *(continued)*
Minerals

- Are inorganic substances that play important roles in:
  - enzyme metabolism
  - membrane transfer of essential compounds
  - regulation of acid-base balance
  - osmotic pressure
  - muscle contractility
  - nerve impulse transmission
  - growth
- Reside in bones, hemoglobin, thyroxine, teeth, and organs
- Are classified as *major minerals* (more than 0.005% of body weight) or *trace minerals* (less than 0.005% of body weight)

Major minerals	Trace minerals
• Calcium	• Chromium
• Chloride	• Cobalt
• Magnesium	• Copper
• Phosphorus	• Fluorine
• Potassium	• Iodine
• Sodium	• Iron
	• Manganese
	• Molybdenum
	• Selenium
	• Zinc

Remember to take in all of your minerals— even the trace ones— or you'll never grow up to be big and strong like me.

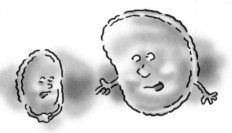

Guide to minerals

Mineral	Major functions
Calcium	Blood clotting, bone and tooth formation, cardiac rhythm, cell membrane permeability, muscle growth and contraction, nerve impulse transmission
Chloride	Maintenance of fluid, electrolyte, acid-base, and osmotic pressure balance
Magnesium	Acid-base balance, metabolism, protein synthesis, muscle relaxation, cellular respiration, nerve impulse transmission
Phosphorus	Bone and tooth formation, cell growth and repair, energy production
Potassium	Cardiac rhythm, muscle contraction, nerve impulse transmission, rapid growth, fluid distribution and osmotic pressure balance, acid-base balance
Sodium	Cellular fluid-level maintenance, muscle contraction, acid-base balance, cell permeability, muscle function, nerve impulse transmission
Fluoride (fluorine)	Bone and tooth formation
Iodine	Thyroid hormone production, energy production, metabolism, physical and mental development
Iron	Growth (in children), hemoglobin production, stress and disease resistance, cellular respiration, oxygen transport
Selenium	Immune mechanisms, mitochondrial adenosine triphosphate synthesis, cellular protection
Zinc	Burn and wound healing, carbohydrate digestion, metabolism (carbohydrate, fat, protein), prostate gland function, reproductive organ growth and development, cell growth

Digestion and absorption

● Nutrients must be digested in the GI tract by enzymes that split large units into smaller ones
● This process is called *hydrolysis*

Carbohydrate digestion and absorption

● Enzymes break down complex carbohydrates
● Monosaccharides (glucose, fructose, and galactose) are absorbed through the intestinal mucosa and then transported through the portal venous system to the liver
● In the liver, enzymes convert fructose and galactose to glucose
● Ribonucleases and deoxyribonucleases break down nucleotides from deoxyribonucleic acid and ribonucleic acid into pentoses and nitrogen bases, which are absorbed through the intestinal mucosa

Protein digestion and absorption

● Enzymes digest proteins by hydrolyzing the peptide bonds that link the amino acids of the protein chains
● The process of hydrolyzation restores water molecules
● Intestinal mucosal peptidases break down peptides into their constituent amino acids
● After being absorbed through the intestinal mucosa by active transport mechanisms, these amino acids travel through the portal venous system to the liver
● The liver converts the amino acids not needed for protein synthesis into glucose

(Text continues on page 268.)

Carbohydrate digestion and absorption

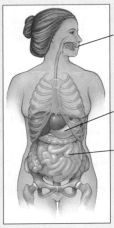

Organ	Action
Mouth	• Chewing breaks down food into smaller particles. • The salivary enzyme amylase acts on starch to break it down first into dextrins and then into maltose.
Stomach	• Peristalsis mixes food particles with gastric secretions.
Small intestine	• The pancreatic enzyme amylase continues the breakdown of starch to maltose. • The intestinal enzyme sucrase acts on sucrose to produce fructose. • The intestinal enzyme lactase acts on lactose to produce galactose. • The intestinal enzyme maltase acts on maltose to produce glucose.

Enzymes active in protein digestion

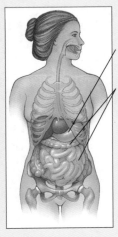

Organ	Active enzymes	Digestive action
Stomach	Pepsin	Breaks protein into polypeptides
Intestine	Trypsin-pancreatic enzyme	Breaks protein and polypeptides into tripeptides and dipeptides
	Chymotrypsin-pancreatic enzyme	Breaks protein and polypeptides into tripeptides and dipeptides
	Carboxypeptidase	Breaks polypeptides into simpler peptides and amino acids
	Aminopeptidase	Breaks polypeptides into peptides, dipeptides, and amino acids
	Dipeptidase	Breaks dipeptides into amino acids

Digestion and absorption *(continued)*
Lipid digestion and absorption

- Pancreatic lipase breaks down fats and phospholipids into a mixture of glycerol, short- and long-chain fatty acids, and monoglycerides
- Fat enters the duodenum in a congealed mass
  - The gallbladder releases bile to emulsify the fat
  - This allows lipase to accelerate its digestion of the fat
- Fat is absorbed through the villi of the small intestines
- Glycerol diffuses directly through the intestinal mucosa
- Short-chain fatty acids are absorbed into the bloodstream via intestinal capillaries and then carried to the liver by the portal venous system
- Long-chain fatty acids and monoglycerides are absorbed into the fatty walls of the villi and changed into triglycerides
  - Triglycerides are coated with cholesterol and protein, forming *chylomicrons*
  - Chylomicrons enter a lacteal and are carried through the lymphatic channels to the thoracic duct
  - From the thoracic duct, they enter the bloodstream
  - They're then broken down into fatty acids and glycerol, after which they're absorbed and recombined in fat cells, reforming triglycerides for storage and later use

Fat digestion and absorption

1.

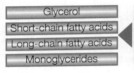

Pancreatic lipase

Glycerol
Short-chain fatty acids
Long-chain fatty acids
Monoglycerides

Fats, phospholipids

2.

Gallbladder

Congealed mass of fat

Duodenum

Fat entering duodenum

3.

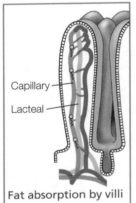

Capillary

Lacteal

Fat absorption by villi

4.

Long-chain fatty acid

Triglycerides synthesized

Formation of chylomicrons

Lacteal

Monoglyceride

Passage of chylomicrons to lacteal

Absorption of long-chain fatty acids and monoglycerides

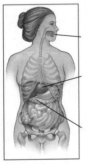

Organ	Active enzymes	Digestive action
Mouth	• Lingual lipase	Minimal amount of fat digestion
Liver	• Bile	Prepares fat for absorption by breaking it into tiny particles (emulsification)
Pancreas	• Pancreatic lipase	Breaks down fats into fatty acids and glycerol

Metabolism

- Is the process by which food substances are transformed into energy or materials that the body can use or store
- Involves two processes:
  - *anabolism*—synthesis of simple substances into complex ones
  - *catabolism*—breakdown of complex substances into simpler ones or into energy

Carbohydrate metabolism

- All ingested carbohydrates are converted to glucose, the body's main energy source
- Glucose catabolism generates energy in three phases: glycolysis, Krebs cycle, and the electron transport chain

Glycolysis

- Enzymes break down one molecule of glucose to form pyruvate
- Pyruvate yields energy in the form of ATP and acetyl CoA

Krebs cycle

- A molecule of acetyl CoA is oxidized by enzymes to yield energy
- Fragments of acetyl CoA join to oxaloacetic acid to form citric acid
- The CoA molecule detaches from the acetyl group to form more acetyl CoA molecules
- Enzymes convert citric acid into intermediate compounds and then back into oxaloacetic acid
- The process also liberates carbon dioxide

Electron-transport chain

- Molecules on the inner mitochondrial membrane pick up electrons from the hydrogen atoms and transport them through oxidation-reduction reactions in the mitochondria
- The hydrogen ions produced in the Krebs cycle combine with oxygen to form water

(Text continues on page 272.)

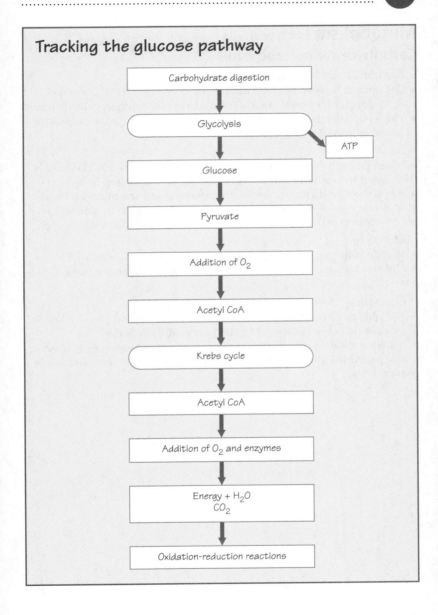

Metabolism *(continued)*

Carbohydrate metabolism *(continued)*

Regulation of blood glucose levels

- Because all ingested carbohydrates are converted to glucose, the body depends on certain organ systems to regulate blood glucose levels
- The liver, the muscles, and hormones all play a role in the regulation of blood glucose levels

Liver

- When glucose levels exceed the body's immediate needs, the liver is stimulated by hormones to convert glucose into glycogen or lipids
- When the blood glucose levels drop excessively, the liver can form glucose by *glycogenolysis* (the breakdown of glycogen to glucose) and *gluconeogenesis* (the synthesis of glucose from amino acids)

Muscle cells

- Muscle cells can convert glucose to glycogen for storage
- Muscles lack the enzymes necessary to convert glycogen back to glucose

Hormones

- The only hormone that can significantly reduce blood glucose levels is *insulin,* which is produced by the pancreatic islet cells
- Insulin promotes cell uptake and use of glucose as an energy source; it also promotes glucose storage as glycogen (*glycogenesis*) and lipids (*lipogenesis*)

(Text continues on page 274.)

The liver's role in the regulation of blood glucose levels

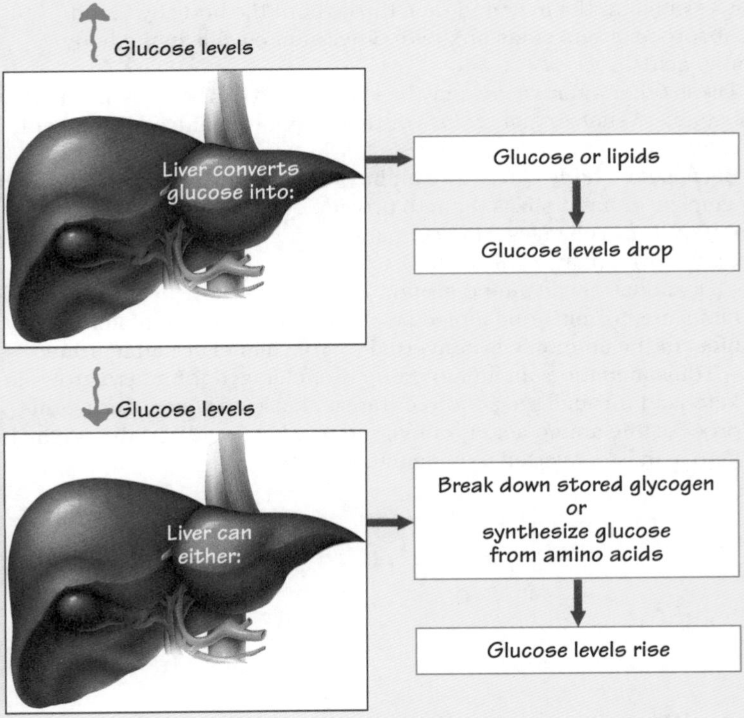

Glucose levels

Liver converts glucose into:

Glucose or lipids

Glucose levels drop

Glucose levels

Liver can either:

Break down stored glycogen
or
synthesize glucose
from amino acids

Glucose levels rise

Metabolism *(continued)*

Protein metabolism

● Proteins are absorbed as amino acids and carried by the portal venous system to the liver and then throughout the body by blood
● Absorbed amino acids mix with other amino acids in the body's amino acid pool
● These other amino acids may be synthesized by the body from other substances (such as *keto acids*) or they may be produced by protein breakdown
● Because the body can't store amino acids, it converts them to protein or glucose or catabolizes them to provide energy
● Before these changes can occur, amino acids must be transformed by *deamination* or *transamination*
  – Deamination: an amino group ($-NH_2$) splits off from an amino acid molecule, forming one molecule of ammonia and one of keto acid; most of the ammonia is converted to urea and excreted in urine
  – Transamination: an amino group is exchanged for a keto group in a keto acid through the action of transaminase enzymes; during this process, the amino acid is converted to a keto acid and the original keto acid is converted to an amino acid

(Text continues on page 276.)

Protein metabolism

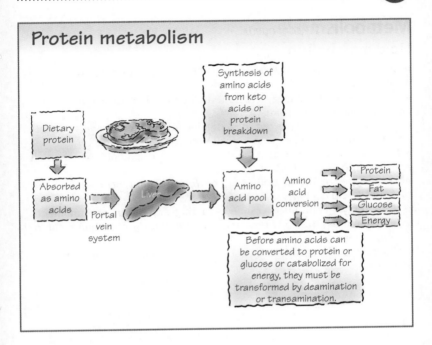

Metabolism *(continued)*
Lipid metabolism

- Lipids are stored in adipose tissue within cells until they're required for use as fuel
- When needed for energy, each fat molecule is hydrolyzed to glycerol and three molecules of fatty acids
- Glycerol can be converted to pyruvic acid and then to acetyl CoA, which enters the Krebs cycle
- Fatty acid catabolism also yields acetyl CoA fragments, which the liver forms into ketone bodies
- Three types of ketone bodies are *acetoacetic acid, beta-hydroxybutyric acid,* and *acetone*
- Under certain conditions (such as fasting, starvation, and uncontrolled diabetes) the body produces more ketone bodies than it can oxidize for energy
- The body must then use fat, rather than glucose, as its primary energy source

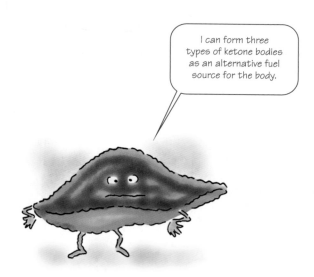

I can form three types of ketone bodies as an alternative fuel source for the body.

Lipid metabolism

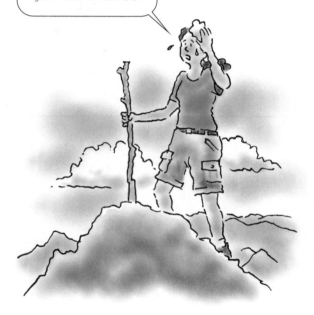

14

Urinary system

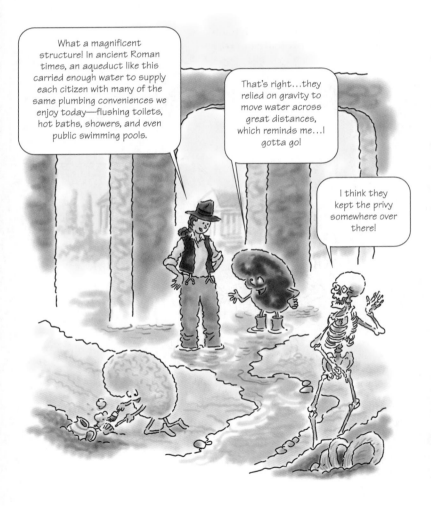

Structures of the urinary system

- The urinary system consists of:
  - two kidneys
  - two ureters
  - bladder
  - urethra
- It functions to:
  - remove wastes from the body
  - help maintain acid-base balance by retaining and excreting hydrogen ions
  - regulate fluid and electrolyte balance
  - assist in blood pressure control

As you can see by the illustration of the male urinary system on the next page, the right kidney extends lower than the left because of the space taken up by the liver. Consequently, the right ureter is shorter than the left one.

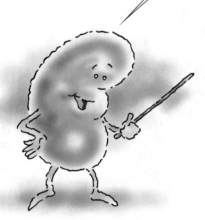

(Text continues on page 282.)

Components of the male urinary system

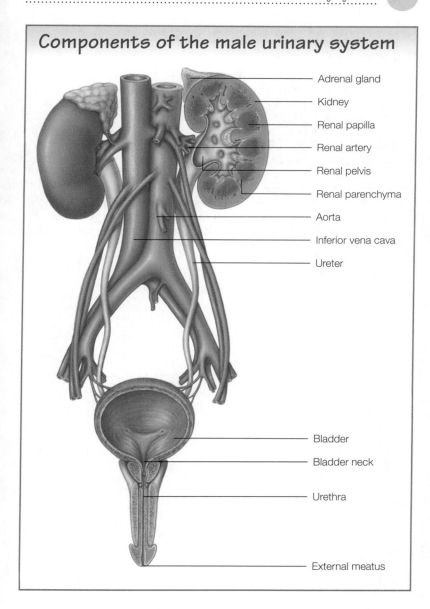

Adrenal gland

Kidney

Renal papilla

Renal artery

Renal pelvis

Renal parenchyma

Aorta

Inferior vena cava

Ureter

Bladder

Bladder neck

Urethra

External meatus

Structures of the urinary system *(continued)*
Kidneys
- Are bean-shaped, highly vascular organs
- Consist of three regions:
  - *Renal cortex* (outer region): contains blood-filtering mechanisms and is protected by a fibrous capsule and layers of fat
  - *Renal medulla* (middle region): contains 8 to 12 renal pyramids (striated wedges that are composed mostly of tubular structures)
  - *Renal pelvis* (inner region): receives urine through the major calyces
- Supports the adrenal glands; one gland lies on top of each kidney
  - These glands are affected by the release of renin from the kidneys
  - In turn, the adrenal glands affect the renal system by influencing blood pressure as well as sodium and water retention in the kidneys

(Text continues on page 284.)

Kidney regions

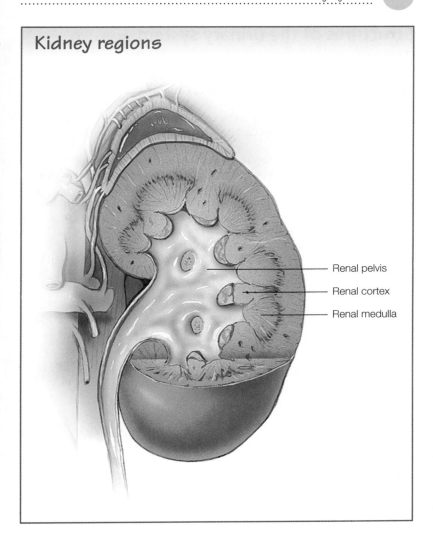

— Renal pelvis

— Renal cortex

— Renal medulla

Structures of the urinary system *(continued)*
Kidneys *(continued)*

- Protected anteriorly by the contents of the abdomen and posteriorly by the muscles attached to the vertebral column
- Have many functions, including:
  - the elimination of wastes and excess ions (in the form of urine)
  - blood filtration (by regulating chemical composition and blood volume)
  - maintenance of fluid-electrolyte and acid-base balances
  - production and release of renin to promote angiotensin II activation and aldosterone production in the adrenal gland
  - production of erythropoietin (a hormone that stimulates red blood cell [RBC] production) and enzymes (such as renin, which governs blood pressure and kidney function)
  - conversion of vitamin D to a more active form

(Text continues on page 286.)

The kidneys

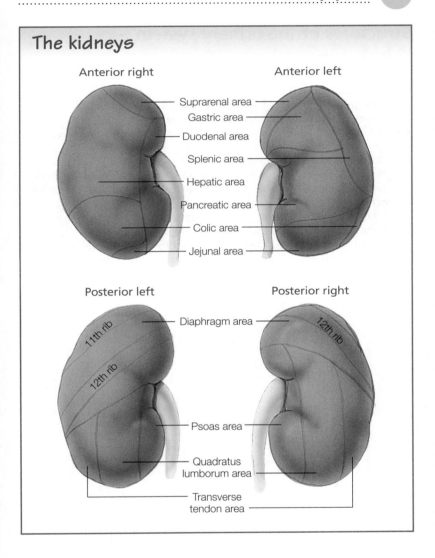

Anterior right

Anterior left

- Suprarenal area
- Gastric area
- Duodenal area
- Splenic area
- Hepatic area
- Pancreatic area
- Colic area
- Jejunal area

Posterior left

Posterior right

11th rib

12th rib

12th rib

- Diaphragm area
- Psoas area
- Quadratus lumborum area
- Transverse tendon area

Structures of the urinary system *(continued)*

Kidneys *(continued)*

The nephron

- Has two main functions:
  - Filtering fluids, wastes, electrolytes, acids, and bases
  - Selectively reabsorbing and secreting ions
- Consists of a cluster of capillaries called a *glomerulus* and a collecting duct
- Is divided into three main portions:
  - *Proximal convoluted tubule*: circulates water and reabsorbs glucose, amino acids, metabolites, and electrolytes from the filtrate into nearby capillaries
  - *Loop of Henle*: concentrates the filtrate through electrolyte exchange and reabsorption to produce a hyperosmolar fluid
  - *Distal convoluted tubule*: point where filtrate enters the collecting tubule and where sodium is reabsorbed under the influence of aldosterone

> The nephron is my basic functional unit. It filters fluids, wastes, electrolytes, acids, and bases and it selectively reabsorbs and secretes ions. Pretty cool, huh!

(Text continues on page 288.)

The nephron

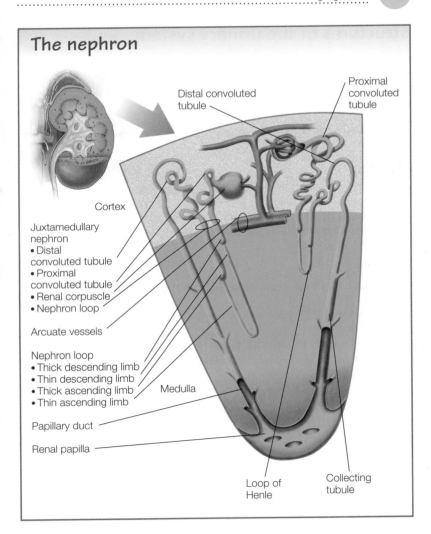

Distal convoluted tubule

Proximal convoluted tubule

Cortex

Juxtamedullary nephron
• Distal convoluted tubule
• Proximal convoluted tubule
• Renal corpuscle
• Nephron loop

Arcuate vessels

Nephron loop
• Thick descending limb
• Thin descending limb
• Thick ascending limb
• Thin ascending limb

Medulla

Papillary duct

Renal papilla

Loop of Henle

Collecting tubule

Structures of the urinary system (continued)
Ureters

- Are fibromuscular tubes that connect each kidney to the bladder (with the left ureter being slightly longer than the right)
- Are surrounded by a three-layered wall
- Act as conduits that carry urine from the kidneys to the bladder
- Have peristaltic waves one to five times each minute to channel urine toward the bladder

Bladder

- Is a hollow, sphere-shaped, muscular organ in the pelvis
- Functions to store urine
- Has a capacity of 500 to 600 ml in a normal adult
- Has three openings in its base that form a triangular area called the *trigone*

Urethra

- Is a small duct that channels urine from the bladder to the outside of the body
- Is embedded in the anterior wall of the vagina behind the symphysis pubis in females
- Passes vertically through the *prostate* gland and then extends through the urogenital diaphragm and penis in males

Male ureters, bladder, and urethra

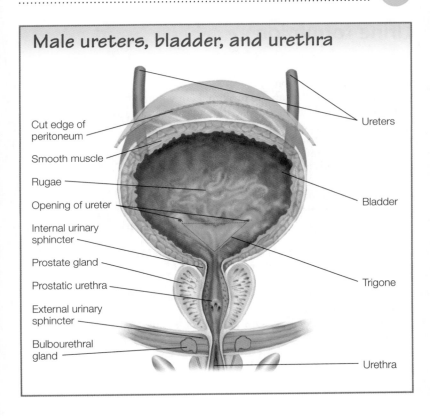

Cut edge of peritoneum

Smooth muscle

Rugae

Opening of ureter

Internal urinary sphincter

Prostate gland

Prostatic urethra

External urinary sphincter

Bulbourethral gland

Ureters

Bladder

Trigone

Urethra

Urine formation

- Results from three processes that occur in the nephrons: glomerular filtration, tubular reabsorption, and tubular secretion
- In glomerular filtration:
  - active transport from the proximal convoluted tubules leads to re-absorption of Na^+ and glucose into nearby circulation
  - osmosis then causes H_2O reabsorption
- In tubular reabsorption:
  - a substance moves from the filtrate back from the distal convoluted tubules, into the peritubular capillaries
  - active transport results in Na^+ reabsorption
  - the presence of ADH causes H_2O reabsorption
- In tubular secretion:
  - A substance moves from the peritubular capillaries into the tubular filtrate
  - peritubular capillaries then secrete NH_3 and H^+
- Typically produces a daily urine output of 720 to 2,400 ml
  - Varies with fluid intake and climate
  - Urine output increases after drinking a large volume of fluid, as the body excretes excess water
  - Urine output decreases if fluid intake is reduced or sodium intake is excessive

How the kidneys form urine

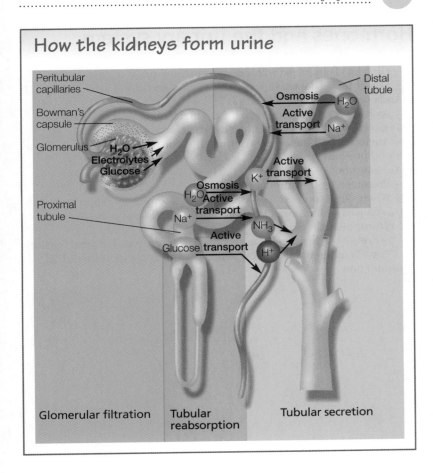

Hormones and the urinary system

- Antidiuretic hormone (ADH)
  - High levels increase water absorption and urine concentration
  - Lower levels decrease water absorption and dilute urine
- Angiotensin I and angiotensin II
  - As it circulates through the lungs, angiotensin I is converted into angiotensin II by angiotensin-converting enzyme
  - Angiotensin II has a constricting effect on the arterioles and raises blood pressure
- Aldosterone
  - Produced by the adrenal cortex
  - When serum potassium levels rise, aldosterone secretion increases; this causes sodium retention, thereby raising blood pressure
- Erythropoietin
  - Secreted by the kidneys in response to low arterial oxygen tension
  - Travels to the bone marrow, where it stimulates increased RBC production

(Text continues on page 294.)

How ADH works

 Low blood volume and increased serum osmolality are sensed by the hypothalamus, which signals the pituitary gland.

 The pituitary gland secretes ADH into the bloodstream.

 ADH causes the kidneys to retain water.

Water retention boosts blood volume and decreases serum osmolality.

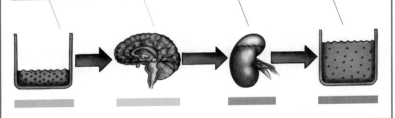

Hormones and the urinary system *(continued)*
Renin-angiotensin-aldosterone system

- Regulates the body's sodium and water levels
- This, in turn, regulates blood pressure
- *Step one*: juxtaglomerular cells near the glomeruli in each kidney secrete the enzyme renin into the blood
- *Step two*: renin circulates throughout the body and converts angiotensin (which is made in the liver) into angiotensin I
- *Step three*: in the lungs, angiotensin I is converted by hydrolysis to angiotensin II
- *Step four*: angiotensin II acts on the adrenal cortex to stimulate production of the hormone aldosterone
- *Step five*: aldosterone acts on the juxtaglomerular cells to increase sodium and water retention and to stimulate or depress further renin secretion, completing the feedback system that automatically readjusts homeostasis

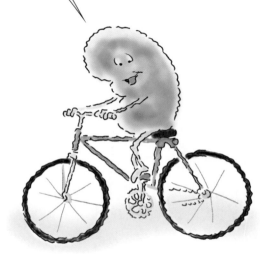

The renin-angiotensin-aldosterone system is a 5-step feedback mechanism that regulates the body's sodium and water levels to help control blood pressure.

Renin-angiotensin-aldosterone system

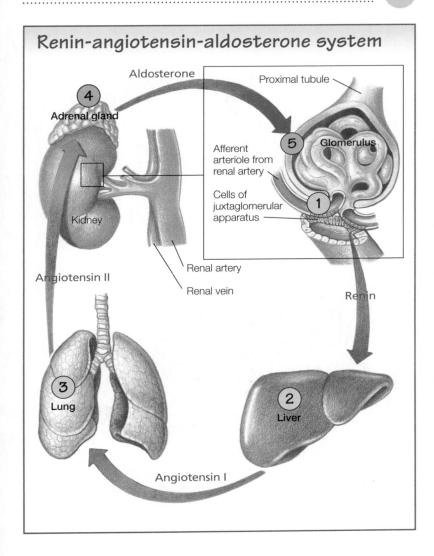

Aldosterone

4
Adrenal gland

Proximal tubule

5 Glomerulus

Afferent
arteriole from
renal artery

Cells of
juxtaglomerular
apparatus

1

Kidney

Angiotensin II

Renal artery

Renal vein

Renin

3
Lung

2
Liver

Angiotensin I

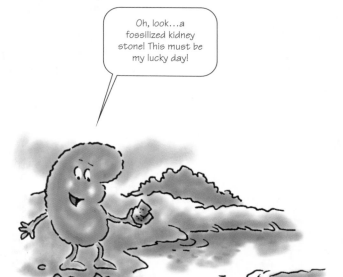

15
Fluids, electrolytes, acids, and bases

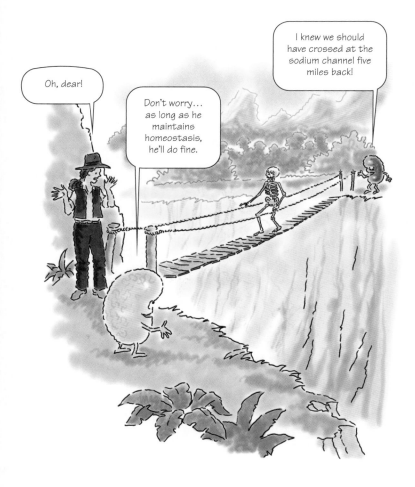

Fluid balance

- The health and *homeostasis* (equilibrium of the various body functions) of the human body depend on *fluid, electrolyte,* and *acid-base balance*
- Factors that disrupt this balance—such as surgery, illness, and injury—can lead to potentially fatal changes in metabolic activity

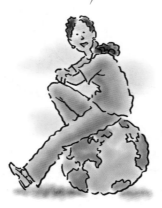

Remember, homeostasis refers to the body's tendency to regulate its internal conditions to stabilize itself despite all the changes going on around it.

(Text continues on page 300.)

Fluid gains and losses

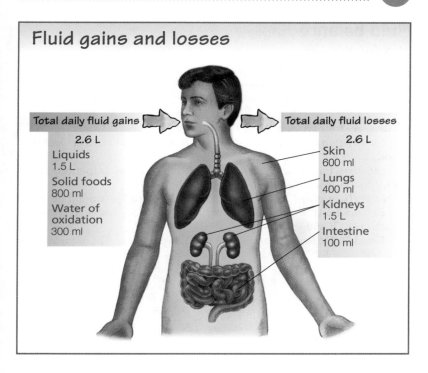

Total daily fluid gains
2.6 L

Liquids
1.5 L

Solid foods
800 ml

Water of
oxidation
300 ml

Total daily fluid losses
2.6 L

Skin
600 ml

Lungs
400 ml

Kidneys
1.5 L

Intestine
100 ml

Fluid balance *(continued)*
The four fluids

● Body fluid consists of water containing solutes: dissolved substances necessary for physiologic functioning

● Solutes include electrolytes, glucose, amino acids, and other nutrients

● There are four types of body fluids:

– *Intracellular fluid (ICF)* is found within the individual cells of the body

– *Intravascular fluid (IVF)*, also known as plasma, is found within the blood vessels and the lymphatic system

– *Interstitial fluid (ISF)* is found in the loose tissue around cells

– *Extracellular fluid (ECF)* is found in the spaces between cells; it includes IVF and ISF

● ICF and ECF comprise about 40% and 20%, respectively, of an adult's total body weight

(Text continues on page 302.)

Body fluids

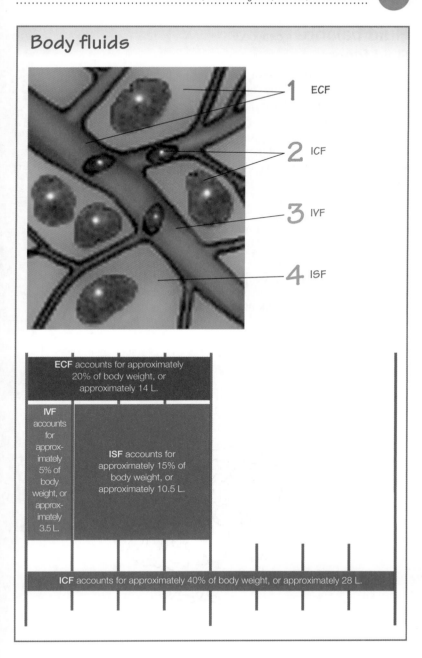

1 ECF

2 ICF

3 IVF

4 ISF

ECF accounts for approximately 20% of body weight, or approximately 14 L.

IVF accounts for approximately 5% of body weight, or approximately 3.5 L.

ISF accounts for approximately 15% of body weight, or approximately 10.5 L.

ICF accounts for approximately 40% of body weight, or approximately 28 L.

Fluid balance (continued)
Fluid forms

- Fluids in the body generally aren't found in pure forms
- They're most commonly found in three types of solutions: *isotonic*, *hypotonic*, and *hypertonic*

Isotonic solution
- Has the same solute concentration as another solution
- No imbalance means no net fluid shift
- Cells won't shrink or swell because there's no gain or loss of water in the cell

Hypotonic solution
- Has a lower solute concentration than another solution
- Administration of a hypotonic solution would cause water to move into the cells, making them swell

Hypertonic solution
- Has a higher solute concentration than another solution
- Administration of a hypertonic solution would cause water to be drawn out of the cells, making them shrink

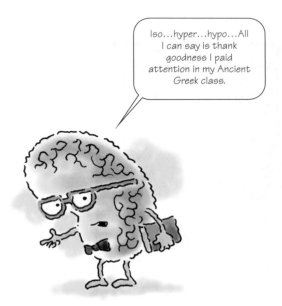

Iso...hyper...hypo...All I can say is thank goodness I paid attention in my Ancient Greek class.

(Text continues on page 304.)

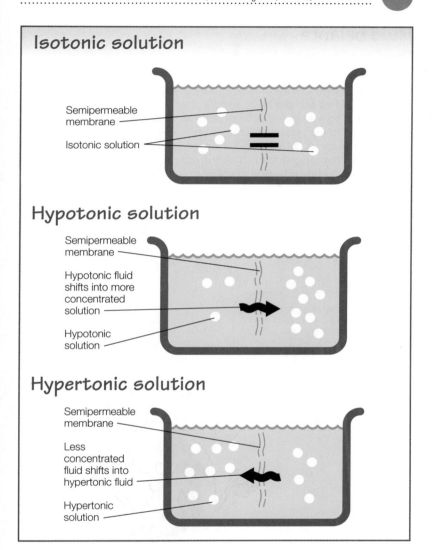

Isotonic solution

Semipermeable
membrane

Isotonic solution

Hypotonic solution

Semipermeable
membrane

Hypotonic fluid
shifts into more
concentrated
solution

Hypotonic
solution

Hypertonic solution

Semipermeable
membrane

Less
concentrated
fluid shifts into
hypertonic fluid

Hypertonic
solution

Fluid balance (continued)

Fluid movement within cells

- Fluids and solutes move constantly within the body
- That movement allows the body to maintain *homeostasis* (the constant state of balance the body seeks)
- *Diffusion*: movement of solutes from an area of high concentration to an area of lower concentration
- *Active transport*: solutes move from an area of lower concentration to an area of higher concentration; the energy required for solutes to move against a concentration gradient comes from adenosine triphosphate (ATP)
- *Osmosis*: passive movement of fluid from an area of lower solute concentration (and comparatively more fluid) into an area of higher solute concentration (and comparatively less fluid)

Keep your eye on the ball, now...solutes move in diffusion and active transport, and fluid moves in osmosis.

(Text continues on page 306.)

Diffusion

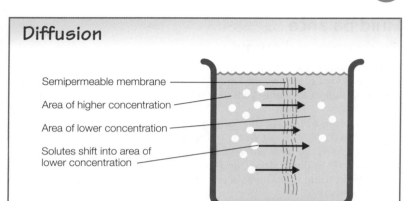

Semipermeable membrane

Area of higher concentration

Area of lower concentration

Solutes shift into area of lower concentration

Active transport

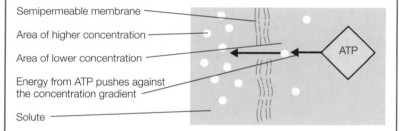

Semipermeable membrane

Area of higher concentration

Area of lower concentration

Energy from ATP pushes against the concentration gradient

Solute

ATP

Osmosis

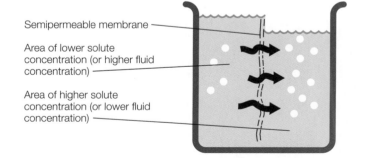

Semipermeable membrane

Area of lower solute concentration (or higher fluid concentration)

Area of higher solute concentration (or lower fluid concentration)

Fluid balance (continued)

Fluid intake and output

- Water normally enters the body from the GI tract
  - The body obtains about 1.6 qt (1.5 L) of water from consumed liquids and approximately 26.6 oz (800 ml) more from solid foods each day
  - Oxidation of food in the body yields carbon dioxide (CO_2) and about 10 oz (300 ml) of water (water of oxidation)
- Water leaves the body through the skin (in perspiration), lungs (in expired air), GI tract (in stool), and urinary tract (in urine)
- The main route of water loss is urine excretion (which varies from 1 to 2.6 L daily)
- Water losses through the skin (600 ml) and lungs (400 ml) amount to 1 L daily but may increase markedly with strenuous exertion, which predisposes a person to dehydration
- Fluid gains should match fluid losses to maintain proper physiologic functioning
- Interruption or dysfunction of one or both of the mechanisms that regulate fluid balance—thirst and the *countercurrent mechanism* (fluid regulation by the kidneys)—can lead to a fluid imbalance

Maintaining fluid balance

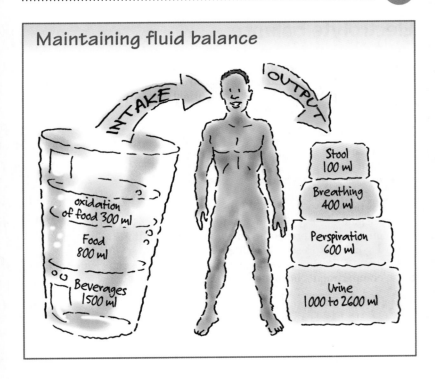

INTAKE

OUTPUT

oxidation of food 300 ml

Food 800 ml

Beverages 1500 ml

Stool 100 ml

Breathing 400 ml

Perspiration 600 ml

Urine 1000 to 2600 ml

Electrolyte balance

- *Electrolytes*: substances that *dissociate* (break up) into electrically charged particles, called *ions*, when dissolved in water
- Adequate amounts of each major electrolyte and a proper balance of electrolytes are required to maintain normal physiologic functioning
- *Cations* (positively charged ions) include:
  - sodium
  - potassium
  - calcium
  - magnesium
- *Anions* (negatively charged ions) include:
  - chloride
  - bicarbonate
  - phosphate
- Because ions are present in such low concentrations in body fluids, they're usually expressed in milliequivalents per liter (mEq/L)
- ICF and ECF cells are permeable to different substances; therefore, these compartments normally have different electrolyte compositions

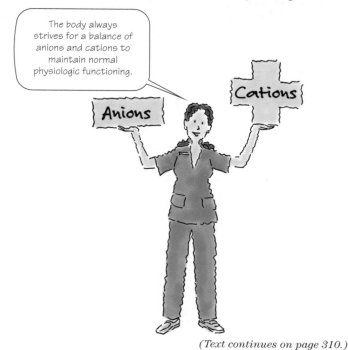

The body always strives for a balance of anions and cations to maintain normal physiologic functioning.

Anions

Cations

(Text continues on page 310.)

Electrolyte composition in ICF and ECF

Electrolyte	ICF	ECF
Sodium	10 mEq/L	136 to 146 mEq/L
Potassium	140 mEq/L	3.6 to 5 mEq/L
Calcium	10 mEq/L	4.5 to 5.8 mEq/L
Magnesium	40 mEq/L	1.6 to 2.2 mEq/L
Chloride	4 mEq/L	96 to 106 mEq/L
Bicarbonate	10 mEq/L	24 to 28 mEq/L
Phosphate	100 mEq/L	1 to 1.5 mEq/L

Electrolyte balance *(continued)*

Electrolyte regulatory mechanisms

- The kidneys and aldosterone are the chief sodium regulators
  - The small intestine absorbs sodium readily from food
  - The skin and kidneys excrete sodium
- The kidneys also regulate potassium
  - This is done through the action of aldosterone
  - Most potassium is absorbed from food in the GI tract
- Parathyroid hormone (PTH) is the main regulator of calcium
  - Controls calcium uptake from the GI tract
  - Also controls calcium excretion by the kidneys
- Magnesium is governed by aldosterone
  - Aldosterone controls renal magnesium reabsorption
  - Absorbed from the GI tract, magnesium is excreted in urine, breast milk, and saliva
- The kidneys also regulate chloride, which moves in conjunction with sodium ions
- The kidneys regulate bicarbonate
  - Kidneys excrete, absorb, and form bicarbonate
  - Bicarbonate plays a vital part in acid-base balance
- The kidneys regulate phosphate
  - Absorbed from food, phosphate is incorporated with calcium in bone
  - PTH governs calcium and phosphate levels

Osmotic regulation of sodium and water

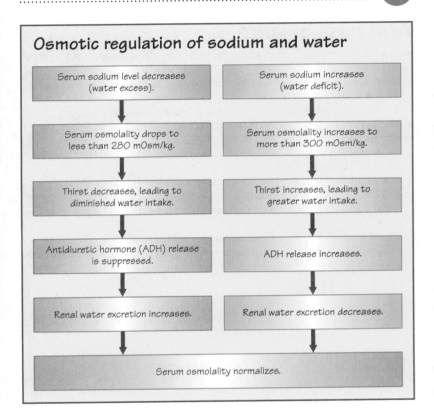

Acid-base balance

- *Acid*: a substance that yields hydrogen ions when dissociated in solution
- *Base*: a substance that dissociates in water, releasing ions that can combine with hydrogen ions
- A neutral solution, such as pure water, dissociates only slightly
- The hydrogen ion concentration of a fluid determines whether it's acidic or basic (alkaline)
    - An acidic solution contains more hydrogen (H^+) ions than hydroxide (OH^-) ions; its pH is less than 7
    - A neutral solution contains equal amounts of H^+ and OH^- ions; a pH of 7 indicates neutrality
    - An alkaline solution contains more OH^- ions than H^+ ions; its pH exceeds 7
- Blood pH stays within a narrow range: 7.35 to 7.45
- This acid-base balance is maintained by buffer systems and the lungs and kidneys, which neutralize and eliminate acids as rapidly as they're formed

(Text continues on page 314.)

Maintaining acid-base balance

	pH	Examples
Acidic H^+	0	Hydrochloric acid
	1	Stomach acid
	2	Lemon juice
	3	Vinegar, cola, beer
	4	Tomatoes
	5	Black coffee
	6	Urine
	6.5	Saliva
Neutral	7	Distilled water, ICF
	7.4	Arterial blood
	8	Sea water
	9	Baking soda
	10.0	Great Salt Lake
	11	Household ammonia
	12	Bicarbonate of soda
	13	Oven cleaner
Basic (alkaline) OH^-	14	Sodium hydroxide

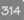

Acid-base balance *(continued)*

Acidosis

- Causes blood pH to fall below 7.35
- May be respiratory or metabolic

Respiratory acidosis

- Occurs when pulmonary ventilation decreases
- Causes CO_2 to be retained, leading to $Paco_2$ levels above 45 mm Hg
- Blood pH level falls below 7.35
- Signs and symptoms include:
  - decreased arterial oxygen saturation
  - rapid, shallow respirations
  - cerebral edema and depressed CNS activity
  - depressed cardiac functions

Metabolic acidosis

- Results when H ions accumulate in the body
- Causes the pH level to fall
- The respiratory rate increases to compensate
- Blood pH level eventually falls below 7.35
- The HCO_3^- level falls below 22 mEq/L
- Signs and symptoms include hyperkalemia and progressive CNS depression

(Text continues on page 316.)

Respiratory acidosis

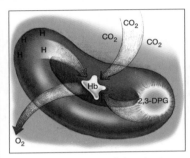

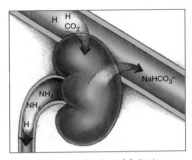

As the pH level falls, 2,3-diphosphoglycerate (2,3-DPG) increases in the red blood cells and causes a change in hemoglobin (Hb) that makes the Hb release oxygen (O_2). The altered Hb, now strongly alkaline, picks up H ions and CO_2, thus eliminating some of the free H ions and excess CO_2.

As respiratory mechanisms fail, the increasing $Paco_2$ stimulates the kidneys to retain HCO_3^- and sodium (Na) ions and to excrete H ions, some of which are excreted in the form of ammonium (NH_4). The additional HCO_3^- and Na combine to form extra sodium bicarbonate ($NaHCO_3^-$), which is then able to buffer more free H ions.

Metabolic acidosis

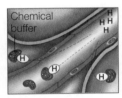

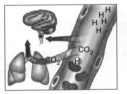

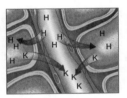

As H ions start to accumulate in the body, chemical buffers (plasma HCO_3^- and proteins) in the cells and ECF bind with them. No signs are detectable at this stage.

Excess H ions (which can't bind with the buffers) decrease the pH and stimulate chemoreceptors in the medulla to increase the respiratory rate. The increased respiratory rate lowers the $Paco_2$, which allows more H ions to bind with HCO_3^- ions. Respiratory compensation occurs within minutes, but isn't sufficient to correct the imbalance.

Excess H ions in the ECF diffuse into cells. To maintain the balance of the charge across the membrane, the cells release K ions into the blood.

Acid-base balance *(continued)*
Alkalosis
- Causes blood pH level to rise above 7.45
- May be respiratory or metabolic

Respiratory alkalosis
- Occurs when pulmonary ventilation increases
- Causes excess CO_2 to be exhaled, leading to a $Paco_2$ level less than 35 mm Hg
- Blood pH level rises above 7.45
- HCO_3^- level falls below 22 mEq/L
- Signs and symptoms include:
  - hypokalemia
  - cerebral vasoconstriction
  - slowing respiratory rate, hypoventilation, Cheyne-Stokes respirations, and periods of apnea
  - increased nerve excitability and muscle contractions

Metabolic alkalosis
- Results when excess HCO_3^- ions accumulate in the body
- Causes the blood pH to rise above 7.45
- HCO_3^- level rises above 26 mEq/L
- Signs and symptoms include:
  - alkaline urine
  - polyuria (initially) and then hypovolemia
  - hypokalemia
  - increased excitability of the CNS and peripheral nervous system

(Text continues on page 318.)

Respiratory alkalosis

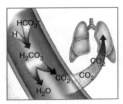

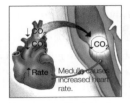

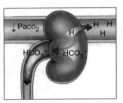

When pulmonary ventilation increases above the amount needed to maintain normal carbon dioxide (CO_2) levels, excessive amounts of CO_2 are exhaled. This leads to a reduction in carbonic acid (H_2CO_3) production, a loss of hydrogen (H) ions and bicarbonate (HCO_3^-) ions, and a subsequent rise in pH.

Hypocapnia stimulates the carotid and aortic bodies and the medulla, which causes an increase in heart rate without an increase in blood pressure.

When hypocapnia lasts more than 6 hours, the kidneys increase secretion of HCO_3^- and reduce excretion of H.

Metabolic alkalosis

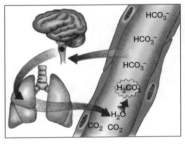

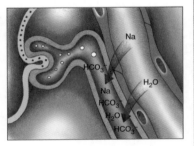

Excess HCO_3^- ions that don't bind with chemical buffers elevate serum pH levels, which, in turn, depress chemoreceptors in the medulla. Depression of those chemoreceptors causes a decrease in respiratory rate, which increases the $Paco_2$. The additional CO_2 combines with H_2O to form H_2CO_3.

To maintain electrochemical balance, the kidneys excrete excess Na ions, H_2O, and HCO_3^-.

Acid-base balance *(continued)*
Buffer systems

● *Buffer systems* reduce the effect of an abrupt change in hydrogen ion concentration by converting a strong acid or base into a weak acid or base

● Buffer systems that help maintain acid-base balance include sodium bicarbonate–carbonic acid, phosphate, and protein

● *Sodium bicarbonate–carbonic acid*: sodium bicarbonate concentration is regulated by the kidneys; carbonic acid concentration is regulated by the lungs

  – The lungs excrete CO_2 and regulate the carbonic acid content of the blood

  – Carbonic acid is derived from the CO_2 and water that are released as by-products of cellular metabolic activity

● *Phosphate*: works by regulating the pH of fluids as they pass through the kidneys

● *Protein*: intracellular proteins absorb hydrogen (H^+) ions generated by the body's metabolic processes and may release excess hydrogen as needed

How respiratory mechanisms affect blood pH

Condition causing decreased blood pH
(such as diabetic acidosis or respiratory depression)

$\downarrow$

Stimulation of respiratory center

$\downarrow$

Increased respiratory rate and depth

$\downarrow$

Decreased blood CO_2 and increased blood pH

$\downarrow$

Normal blood pH

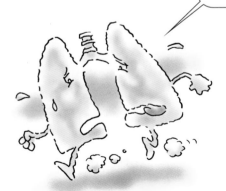

A decrease in blood pH will force me to work harder. All this hard work lowers the blood CO_2 level and, if I've done my job sufficiently, returns the pH to a normal level.

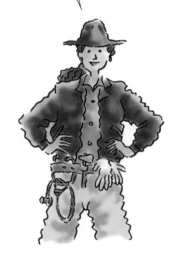

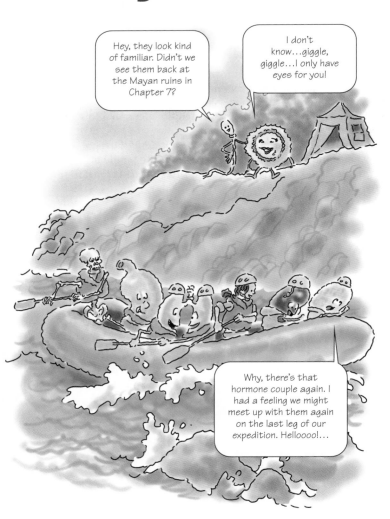

Male reproductive system

- Consists of organs that produce, transfer, and introduce mature sperm into the female reproductive tract, where fertilization occurs
- Also plays a role in secretion of male sex hormones

Penis

- Deposits sperm in the female reproductive tract
- Acts as the terminal duct for the urinary tract
- Consists of an attached root, a free shaft, and the glans penis
- Internally, consists of three columns of *erectile tissue* bound together by *heavy fibrous tissue*
  - Two *corpora cavernosa* form the major part of the penis
  - The *corpus spongiosum* encases the urethra
- Shaft covered by thin, loose skin
- The *urethral meatus* opens through the glans to allow urination and ejaculation
- Receives blood through the *internal pudendal artery*; blood then flows into the corpora cavernosa through the penile artery
- Venous blood returns through the *internal iliac vein* to the *vena cava*

(Text continues on page 324.)

Structures of the male reproductive system

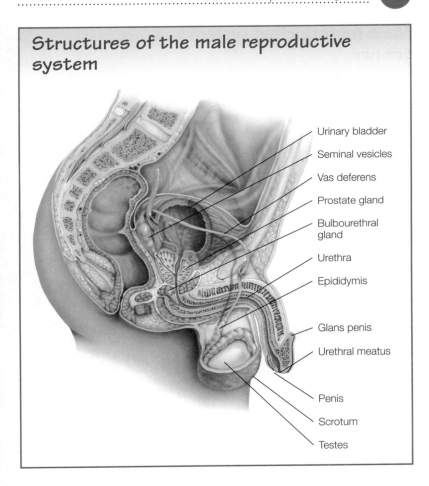

Urinary bladder

Seminal vesicles

Vas deferens

Prostate gland

Bulbourethral gland

Urethra

Epididymis

Glans penis

Urethral meatus

Penis

Scrotum

Testes

Male reproductive system *(continued)*
Scrotum

- Extra-abdominal pouch consisting of a thin layer of skin overlying a tighter, muscle-like layer
- Located posterior to the penis and anterior to the anus
- Meets the penis at the penoscrotal junction
- Muscle-like layer overlies the tunica vaginalis, a serous membrane that covers the internal scrotal cavity
- Internally, divided into two sacs by a *septum*
- Each sac contains a *testis*, an *epididymis*, and a *spermatic cord* (connective tissue sheath that encases autonomic nerve fibers, blood vessels, lymph vessels, and the *vas deferens*)

Testes

- Enveloped in two layers of connective tissue:
    - the *tunica vaginalis* (outer layer)
    - the *tunica albuginea* (inner layer)
- Each testis is separated into lobules
- Each lobule contains one to four *seminiferous tubules*, where spermatogenesis takes place
- Seminiferous tubules are coiled and measure about 29½″ (75 cm) unraveled
- Tubules form a plexus called the *rete testis*

(Text continues on page 326.)

The testes

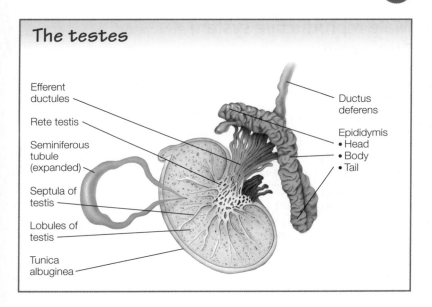

Efferent ductules

Rete testis

Seminiferous tubule (expanded)

Septula of testis

Lobules of testis

Tunica albuginea

Ductus deferens

Epididymis
• Head
• Body
• Tail

Male reproductive system (continued)

Duct system

● Consists of the epididymis, vas deferens, and urethra
● Conveys sperm from the testes to the ejaculatory ducts near the bladder

Epididymis

● A coiled tube located superior to and along the posterior border of the testis
● During ejaculation, smooth muscle in the epididymis contracts, ejecting spermatozoa into the vas deferens

Vas deferens

● Leads from the testes to the abdominal cavity, where it extends upward through the *inguinal canal*, arches over the urethra, and descends behind the bladder
● Has an enlarged portion, called the *ampulla*, that merges with the duct of the seminal vesicle to form the short ejaculatory duct
● After passing through the prostate gland, the vas deferens joins with the urethra

Urethra

● A small tube leading from the floor of the bladder to the exterior
● Consists of three parts: *prostatic urethra*, *membranous urethra*, and *spongy urethra*

(Text continues on page 328.)

The duct system

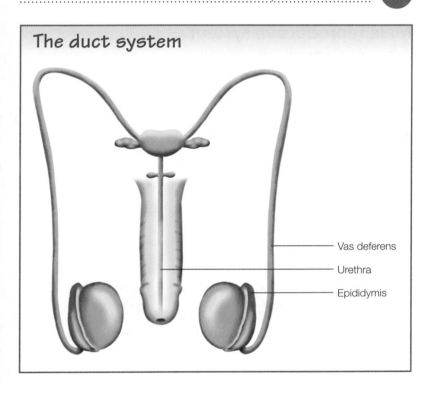

Vas deferens
Urethra
Epididymis

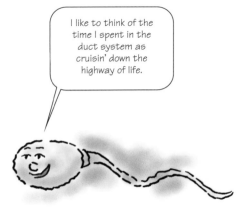

I like to think of the time I spent in the duct system as cruisin' down the highway of life.

Male reproductive system *(continued)*
Accessory reproductive glands
- Produce most of the semen
- Include the *seminal vesicles, bulbourethral glands (Cowper's glands),* and the *prostate gland*

Seminal vesicles
- Paired sacs at the base of the bladder
- Produce roughly 60% of the fluid portion of semen

Prostate gland
- A walnut-sized gland lying under the bladder and surrounding the urethra
- Produces about 30% of the fluid portion of semen
- Continuously secretes prostatic fluid
  - A thin, milky, alkaline fluid that adds volume to semen and enhances sperm motility
  - Fluid also may increase the chances for conception by neutralizing the acidity of the man's urethra and the woman's vagina

Bulbourethral glands
- Paired glands that lie inferior to the prostate
- Secrete an alkaline fluid that's important for counteracting the acid present in the male urethra and female vagina
- Produce mucus that lubricates the urethra

(Text continues on page 330.)

Accessory reproductive glands

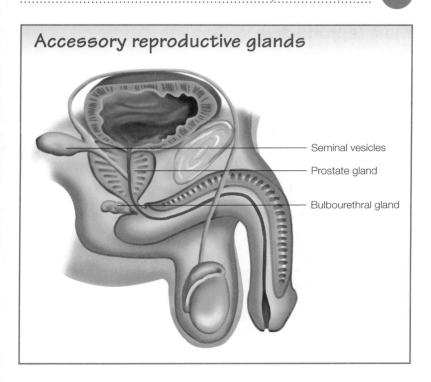

Seminal vesicles

Prostate gland

Bulbourethral gland

Male reproductive system (continued)

Sperm formation

- Called spermatogenesis
- Begins when a male reaches puberty and normally continues throughout life
- Occurs in four stages
- *First*: Primary germinal epithelial cells (called *spermatogonia*) grow and develop into primary *spermatocytes*
  - Both spermatogonia and primary spermatocytes contain 46 chromosomes
  - These consist of 44 *autosomes* and the two sex chromosomes, X and Y
- *Second*: Primary spermatocytes divide to form secondary spermatocytes
  - Each secondary spermatocyte contains one-half the number of autosomes (22)
  - One secondary spermatocyte contains an X chromosome; the other, a Y chromosome
- *Third*: Each secondary spermatocyte divides again to form *spermatids* (also called *spermatoblasts*)
- *Fourth*: Spermatids undergo a series of structural changes that transform them into mature *spermatozoa*, or sperm
  - Each spermatozoon has a head, neck, body, and tail
  - The head contains the *nucleus;* the tail, a large amount of *adenosine triphosphate*, which provides energy for sperm *motility*

(Text continues on page 332.)

Spermatogenesis

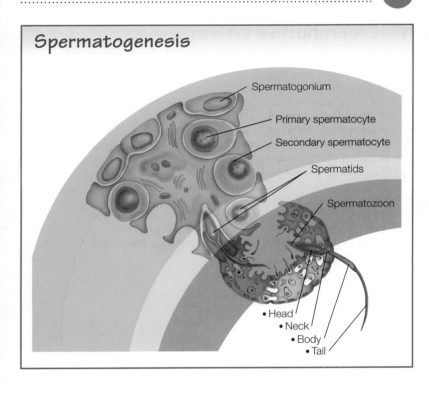

Male reproductive system *(continued)*
Male hormonal control and sexual development

- Male sex hormones, called *androgens*, are produced in the testes and the adrenal glands
- Major androgens include testosterone, luteinizing hormone (LH), and follicle-stimulating hormone (FSH)
- Testosterone is secreted by *Leydig's cells*
  - It's responsible for the development of male sex organs and secondary sex characteristics
  - It's required for spermatogenesis
  - It directly affects sexual differentiation in the fetus
- LH and FSH directly affect secretion of testosterone
- Secretion of gonadotropins from the pituitary gland usually occurs between ages 11 and 14 (marking the onset of puberty)
- These pituitary gonadotropins stimulate testis functioning as well as testosterone secretion

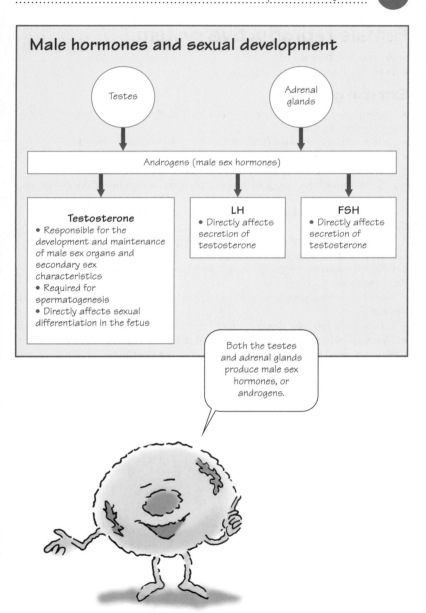

Female reproductive system

- Is largely internal
- Is housed within the pelvic cavity

External genitalia

- *Mons pubis*: a rounded cushion of fatty and connective tissue over the symphysis pubis
- *Labia majora*: extend from the mons pubis to the perineum
- *Labia minora*: lie within and alongside the labia majora
    - Upper section divided into upper and lower lamella
    - Two upper lamellae join to form the *prepuce* (a hoodlike covering over the clitoris)
    - Two lower lamellae form the *frenulum* (the posterior portion of the clitoris)
    - The labia minora contain sebaceous glands, which secrete a lubricant that also acts as a bactericide
- *Clitoris*: contains erectile tissue, venous cavernous spaces, and specialized sensory corpuscles
- *Skene's glands*: produce mucus; located on both sides of the urethral opening
- *Bartholin's glands*: located on either side of the inner vaginal orifice
- *Urethral meatus*: the opening where urine leaves the body
- *Vaginal orifice*: located in the center of the vestibule
- *Perineum*: a complex structure of muscles, blood vessels, fasciae, nerves, and lymphatics located between the lower vagina and the anal canal

(Text continues on page 336.)

Female external genitalia

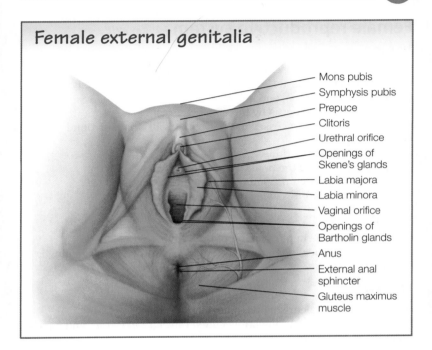

- Mons pubis
- Symphysis pubis
- Prepuce
- Clitoris
- Urethral orifice
- Openings of Skene's glands
- Labia majora
- Labia minora
- Vaginal orifice
- Openings of Bartholin glands
- Anus
- External anal sphincter
- Gluteus maximus muscle

Female reproductive system *(continued)*

Vagina

- Is a highly elastic muscular tube
- Consists of three tissue layers in the vaginal wall: epithelial tissue, loose connective tissue, and muscle tissue
- Connected to the uterus by the uterine cervix
- Has four fornices (recesses in the vaginal wall) that surround the cervix
- Has three main functions:
  - Accommodating the penis during coitus
  - Channeling blood discharged during menstruation
  - Serving as the birth canal during childbirth

Cervix

- Projects into the upper portion of the vagina
- The lower cervical opening is the *external os;* the upper opening is the *internal os*

Uterus

- Is a small, firm, pear-shaped, muscular organ
- Has a mucous membrane lining called the *endometrium,* and a muscular layer called the *myometrium*

(Text continues on page 338.)

Female internal genitalia

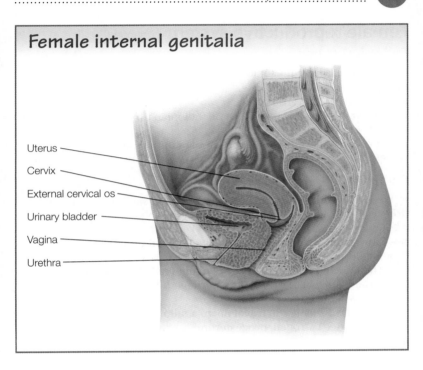

Uterus

Cervix

External cervical os

Urinary bladder

Vagina

Urethra

Female reproductive system *(continued)*

Fallopian tubes

- Are two narrow cylinders of muscle fibers that attach to the uterus at the upper angles of the fundus
- Act as the site of fertilization
- *Ampulla*: the curved portion of the fallopian tube; ends in the funnel-shaped *infundibulum*
- *Fimbriae*: fingerlike projections in the infundibulum that move in waves to sweep the mature ovum from the ovary into the fallopian tube

Ovaries

- Are located on either side of the uterus; their size, shape, and position vary with age
- Each contains approximately 500,000 *graafian follicles* at birth
  - During the childbearing years, one graafian follicle produces an ovum during the first half of each menstrual cycle
  - The follicle releases the mature ovum (called *ovulation*)
  - If the ovum isn't fertilized by sperm within about 1 day from ovulation, it will die
  - If it's fertilized, it will travel down a fallopian tube to the uterus
- Also produce estrogen, progesterone, and a small amount of androgens

(Text continues on page 340.)

Ovaries and fallopian tubes

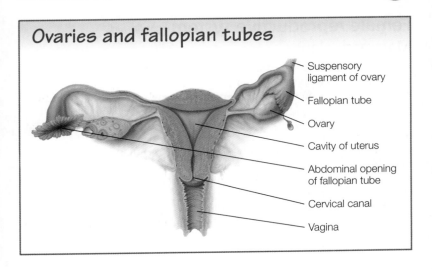

Suspensory ligament of ovary

Fallopian tube

Ovary

Cavity of uterus

Abdominal opening of fallopian tube

Cervical canal

Vagina

Female reproductive system (continued)
Mammary glands

- Are located in the breasts
- Are specialized accessory glands that secrete milk
- Typically function only in the female (although are present in both sexes)
- Contain 15 to 25 lobes separated by fibrous connective tissue and fat in each mammary gland
- Contain clustered *acini*—tiny, saclike duct terminals that secrete milk during lactation—within the lobes
- The ducts draining the gland lobules converge to form excretory (*lactiferous*) ducts and sinuses (*ampullae*)
    - These store milk during lactation
    - These ducts drain onto the nipple surface through 15 to 20 openings

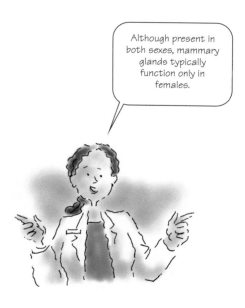

Although present in both sexes, mammary glands typically function only in females.

(Text continues on page 342.)

Mammary glands

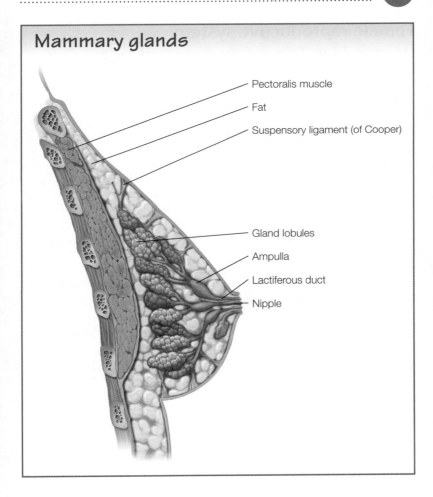

Pectoralis muscle

Fat

Suspensory ligament (of Cooper)

Gland lobules

Ampulla

Lactiferous duct

Nipple

Female reproductive system *(continued)*
Hormonal function and the menstrual cycle
- The female reproductive cycle usually lasts 28 days
- Three different cycles work together: ovarian, hormonal, and endometrial

Ovarian cycle
- The hypothalamus secretes Gn-RH, which stimulates the pituitary gland to secrete FSH and LH
- FSH triggers development of a follicle
- When a follicle matures, LH spikes and the ovum is released
- After ovulation, a corpus luteum forms
- The corpus luteum degenerates if fertilization doesn't occur

Sex hormone cycle
- FSH and LH stimulate estrogen secretion, which peaks just before ovulation
- After ovulation, estrogen levels decline rapidly
- The corpus luteum releases progesterone and estrogen in the luteal phase, then both hormones decline

Endometrial cycle
- The endometrium sheds its functional layer during first 5 days
- It begins regenerating a functional layer at about day 6
- After ovulation, the functional layer becomes the secretory mucosa
- If fertilization doesn't occur, the endometrium sheds its functional layer again

Events in the menstrual cycle

Gonadotropin secretion

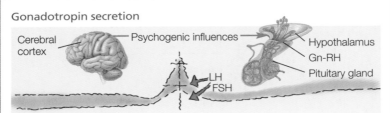

Cerebral cortex — Psychogenic influences — Hypothalamus
Gn-RH
Pituitary gland
LH
FSH

Ovarian cycle

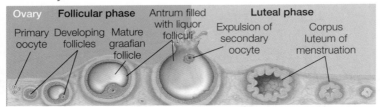

Ovary   **Follicular phase**   Antrum filled with liquor folliculi   **Luteal phase**

Primary oocyte   Developing follicles   Mature graafian follicle   Expulsion of secondary oocyte   Corpus luteum of menstruation

Sex hormone cycle

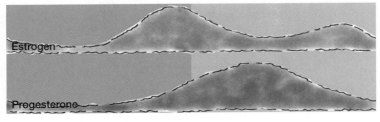

Estrogen

Progesterone

Endometrial (menstrual) cycle

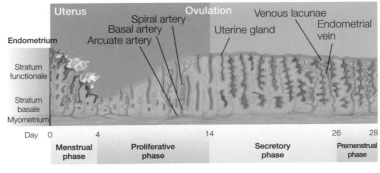

Uterus   Ovulation   Venous lacunae

Spiral artery   Uterine gland   Endometrial vein
Basal artery
Endometrium   Arcuate artery

Stratum functionale

Stratum basale
Myometrium

Day	0	4		14		26	28
		Menstrual phase	Proliferative phase		Secretory phase		Premenstrual phase

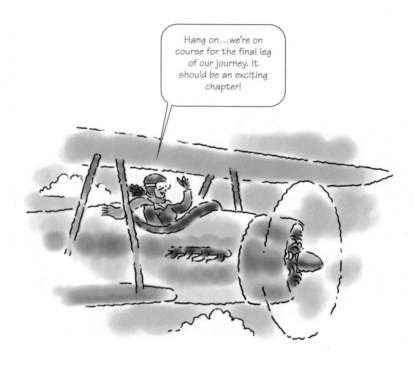

Reproduction and lactation

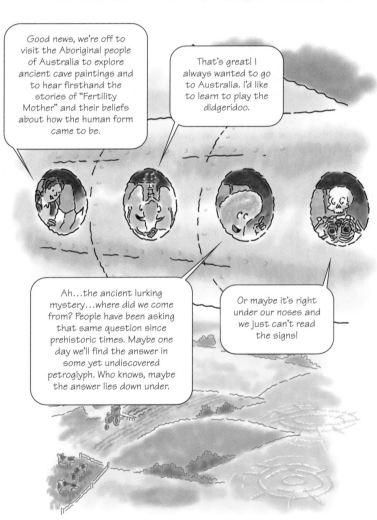

Fertilization

- *Fertilization*: the union of a *spermatozoon* and an *ovum* to form a single cell
- Marks the beginning of the creation of a new human being
- Process involves several steps:
  - First, the spermatozoon, which has a covering called the *acrosome*, approaches the ovum
  - Second, the acrosome develops small perforations through which it releases enzymes necessary for the sperm to penetrate the protective layers of the ovum before fertilization
  - Third, the spermatozoon penetrates the *zona pellucida* (the inner membrane of the ovum); this triggers the ovum's second meiotic division (following meiosis), making the zona pellucida impenetrable to other spermatozoa
  - Fourth, after the spermatozoon penetrates the ovum, its nucleus is released into the ovum, its tail degenerates, and its head enlarges and fuses with the ovum's nucleus
  - This fusion provides the fertilized ovum, called a zygote, with 46 chromosomes

How fertilization occurs

1.

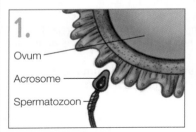

Ovum

Acrosome

Spermatozoon

2.

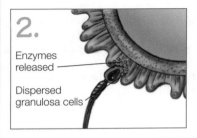

Enzymes released

Dispersed granulosa cells

3.

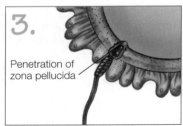

Penetration of zona pellucida

4.

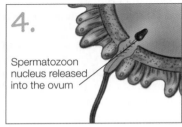

Spermatozoon nucleus released into the ovum

Pregnancy

● Starts with fertilization and ends with childbirth
● Lasts, on average, 38 to 40 weeks
● During this period (called *gestation*), the zygote divides as it passes through the fallopian tube and attaches to the uterine lining via implantation
● A complex sequence of *preembryonic*, *embryonic*, and *fetal* development transforms the zygote into a full-term fetus

Preembryonic development

● Starts with ovum fertilization and lasts for 2 weeks
● Zygote undergoes a series of *mitotic divisions*, or *cleavage*, as it passes through the fallopian tube and it develops into a small mass of cells called a *morula*
● The morula reaches the uterus at or around the 3rd day after fertilization and travels to the uterus
● Now called a *blastocyst*, the structure attaches to the endometrium by the end of the 1st week after fertilization
● During the next week the blastocyst sinks below the endometrium's surface

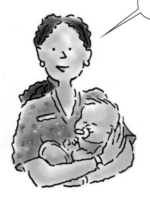

Pregnancy, or the gestational period, lasts about 38 to 40 weeks. It starts with fertilization and ends when the baby is born.

(Text continues on page 350.)

Changes during preembryonic development

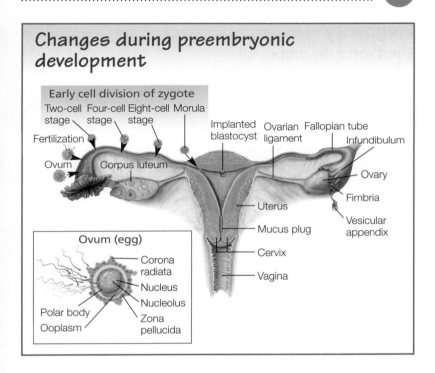

Early cell division of zygote

Two-cell stage · Four-cell stage · Eight-cell stage · Morula

Fertilization

Ovum

Corpus luteum

Implanted blastocyst

Ovarian ligament

Fallopian tube

Infundibulum

Ovary

Fimbria

Uterus

Mucus plug

Vesicular appendix

Cervix

Vagina

Ovum (egg)

Corona radiata

Nucleus

Nucleolus

Polar body

Ooplasm

Zona pellucida

Pregnancy (continued)

Embryonic development

- Occurs during gestational weeks 3 through 8
- The developing zygote is now called an *embryo*
- Each germ layer eventually forms specific tissues in the embryo

Ectoderm

- Epidermis
- Nervous system and pituitary gland
- Salivary glands and tooth enamel
- Optic lens

Mesoderm

- Connective and supporting tissue
- Blood and vascular systems
- Musculature
- Teeth (except enamel)
- Mesothelial lining of the pericardial, pleural, and peritoneal cavities
- Kidneys and ureters

Endoderm

- Pharynx and trachea
- Auditory canal
- Alimentary canal, liver, and pancreas
- Bladder, urethra, and prostate

(Text continues on page 352.)

An embryo

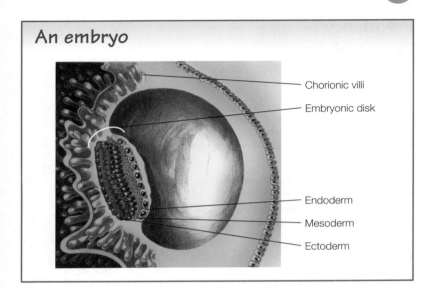

- Chorionic villi
- Embryonic disk
- Endoderm
- Mesoderm
- Ectoderm

Pregnancy *(continued)*
Fetal development
- Lasts from the 9th week until birth
- Maturing fetus enlarges and grows heavier

Month 1
- Head, trunk, and arm and leg buds are discernible
- Cardiovascular system has begun to function
- Primitive form of umbilical cord is visible

Month 2
- Fetus grow to 1″ in length and weighs 1/30 oz
- Head and facial features develop
- External genitalia are present
- Cardiovascular function is complete

Month 3
- Fetus grows to 3″ in length and weighs 1 oz
- Teeth and bones begin to appear and kidneys start to function
- Fetus inhales and exhales amniotic fluid
- Gender is distinguishable

Months 4 to 9
- Fetal growth continues as structures develop rapidly
- Fat and mineral storage occurs

(Text continues on page 354.)

From embryo to fetus

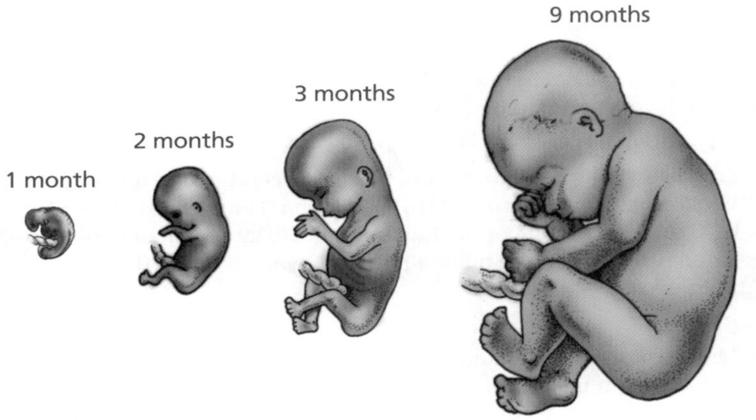

1 month

2 months

3 months

9 months

Pregnancy *(continued)*

Structural changes in the ovaries and uterus

- Pregnancy changes the usual development of the *corpus luteum* (the ovum after ovulation)
- Pregnancy results in the development of the decidua, amniotic sac and fluid, yolk sac, and placenta

Corpus luteum

- Pregnancy stimulates placental tissue to secrete large amounts of human chorionic gonadotropin (HCG), which resembles LH and FSH
- HCG stimulates the corpus luteum to make large amounts of estrogen and progesterone to maintain the pregnancy during the first 3 months

Decidua

- The hormones associated with pregnancy stimulate changes in the endometrial lining, called the *decidua*
- Decidual cells secrete three substances: *prolactin, relaxin,* and *prostaglandin*

Amniotic sac and fluid

- The *amniotic sac*, enclosed within the chorion, gradually enlarges and surrounds the embryo
- The fluid provides the fetus with a buoyant, temperature-controlled environment
- It serves as a fluid wedge that helps open the cervix during birth

(Text continues on page 356.)

Development of the decidua and fetal membranes

Approximately 4 weeks

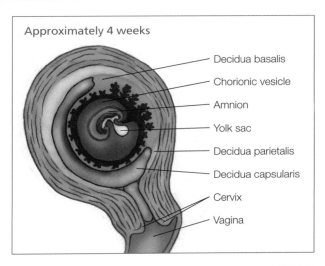

- Decidua basalis
- Chorionic vesicle
- Amnion
- Yolk sac
- Decidua parietalis
- Decidua capsularis
- Cervix
- Vagina

Approximately 16 weeks

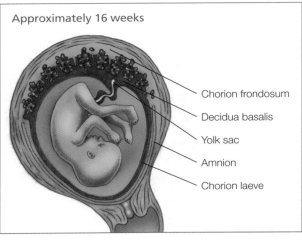

- Chorion frondosum
- Decidua basalis
- Yolk sac
- Amnion
- Chorion laeve

Pregnancy *(continued)*
Structural changes in the ovaries and uterus *(continued)*

Yolk sac
- The *yolk sac* forms next to the endoderm
- A portion of it is incorporated in the developing embryo and forms the GI tract
- Another portion develops into primitive germ cells, which travel to the developing gonads and eventually form *oocytes* or *spermatocytes*

Placenta
- Highly vascular, flattened, disk-shaped organ
- Uses the umbilical cord to provide nutrients to and remove wastes from the fetus from the third month of pregnancy until birth
- The umbilical cord, containing two arteries and one vein, links the fetus to the placenta
  - The umbilical arteries spiral around the cord, divide on the placental surface, and branch off to the chorionic villi
  - Large veins on the surface gather blood returning from the villi and join to form the single umbilical vein, which enters the cord, returning blood to the fetus

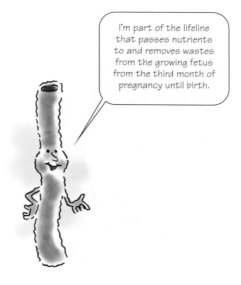

I'm part of the lifeline that passes nutrients to and removes wastes from the growing fetus from the third month of pregnancy until birth.

(Text continues on page 358.)

Placenta

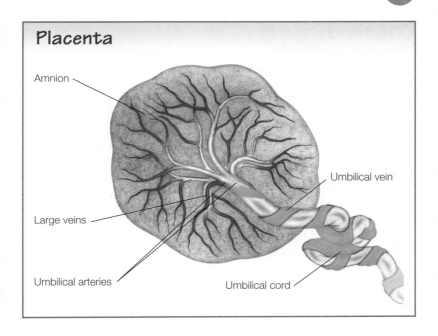

Amnion

Large veins

Umbilical arteries

Umbilical vein

Umbilical cord

Pregnancy *(continued)*
Placental circulation

- Placenta contains two highly specialized circulatory systems
- One system handles uteroplacental circulation and the other handles fetoplacental circulation

Uteroplacental circulation

- Carries oxygenated arterial blood from the maternal circulation to the *intervillous spaces*—large spaces separating chorionic villi in the placenta
- Blood enters the intervillous spaces from uterine arteries that penetrate the basal portion of the placenta
- Blood leaves the intervillous spaces and flows back into the maternal circulation through veins in the basal portion of the placenta near the arteries

Fetoplacental circulation

- Transports oxygen-depleted blood from the fetus to the chorionic villi through the umbilical arteries
- Returns oxygenated blood to the fetus through the umbilical vein

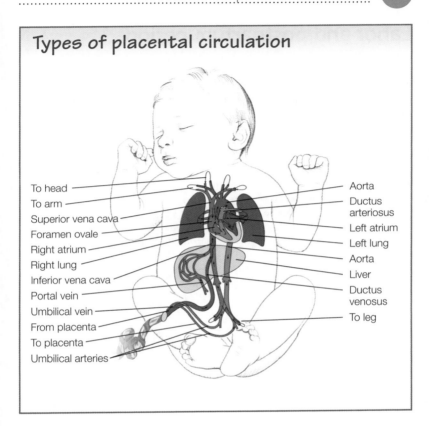

Types of placental circulation

To head

To arm

Superior vena cava

Foramen ovale

Right atrium

Right lung

Inferior vena cava

Portal vein

Umbilical vein

From placenta

To placenta

Umbilical arteries

Aorta

Ductus arteriosus

Left atrium

Left lung

Aorta

Liver

Ductus venosus

To leg

Labor and postpartum period

- *Labor*: the process by which uterine contractions expel the fetus from the uterus
- When labor begins, these contractions become strong and regular
- Eventually, voluntary bearing-down efforts supplement the contractions, resulting in delivery
- The onset of labor results from several factors:
  - An increase is the number of *oxytocin* receptors on uterine muscle fibers
  - Stretching of the uterus over the course of the pregnancy
- Presentation of the fetus takes one of a variety of forms:
  - Cephalic (head-down presentation)
  - Breech (head-up presentation)
  - Shoulder
  - Compound (extremity prolapses alongside major presenting part)

(Text continues on page 362.)

Comparing fetal presentations

Cephalic

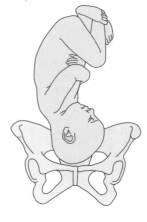

Breech

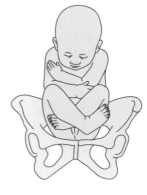

Shoulder

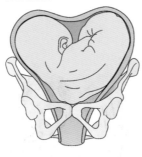

Compound

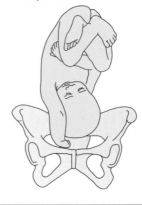

Labor and postpartum period *(continued)*
Stages of labor

● Childbirth can be divided into three stages
● The duration of each stage varies according to the size of the uterus, the woman's age, and the number of previous pregnancies

Stage 1
● The onset of true labor, in which the fetus begins its descent
● Marked by cervical *effacement* (thinning) and *dilation*
● Can last from 6 to 24 hours in primiparous women but is commonly significantly shorter for multiparous women
● Divided into three phases:
  – *Latent phase*: cervix dilates from 0 to 3 cm
  – *Active phase*: cervix dilates from 4 to 7 cm
  – *Transitional phase*: cervix dilates from 8 to 10 cm

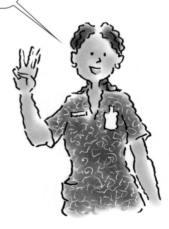

Labor is divided into three distinct stages. The length of each one depends on several factors—the size of the uterus, maternal age, and number of previous pregnancies.

(Text continues on page 364.)

First stage of labor

 Latent phase

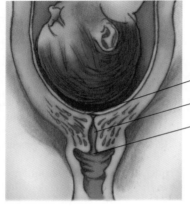

Internal os

Cavity of cervix

External os

No effacement or dilation

 Active phase

Internal os

External os

Early effacement and dilation

 Transitional phase

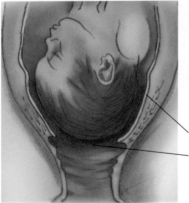

Internal os

External os

Complete effacement and dilation

Labor and postpartum period (continued)
Stages of labor (continued)

Stage 2
- Begins with full cervical dilation and ends with delivery of the fetus
- Averages about 45 minutes in primiparous women; it may be shorter in multiparous women
- Involves rupture of the amniotic sac as uterine contractions increase in frequency and intensity
- As the flexed head of the fetus enters the pelvis, the mother's pelvic muscles force the head to rotate anteriorly and the back of the head to move under the symphysis pubis
- As the uterus contracts, the flexed head of the fetus is forced deeper into the pelvis; resistance of the pelvic floor gradually forces the head to extend
- The head of the fetus rotates back to its former position after passing through the vulvovaginal orifice
- Usually, head rotation is lateral (external) as the anterior shoulder rotates forward to pass under the pubic arch
- Delivery of the shoulders and the rest of the fetus follows

Stage 3
- Starts after childbirth
- Ends with placenta expulsion

Second stage of labor

Internal rotation

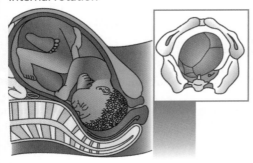

External rotation

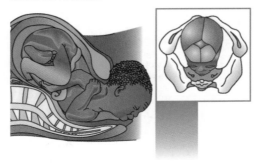

External rotation (shoulder rotation)

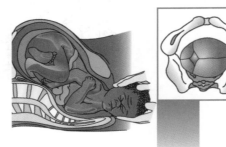

Lactation

- Involves the synthesis of milk and its secretion by the breasts
- Governed by interactions involving estrogen, progesterone, prolactin, and oxytocin
  - First, progesterone and estrogen levels drop, which triggers the production of prolactin
  - Prolactin stimulates milk production by the acinar cells in the mammary glands
  - Milk flows from the acinar cells through small tubules to the lactiferous sinuses
  - When the neonate sucks at the breast, oxytocin is released, causing the nipple to contract and pushing the milk forward through the nipple to the neonate

Milk production is caused by a series of hormonal interactions involving estrogen, progesterone, prolactin, and oxytocin.

Structures used in lactation

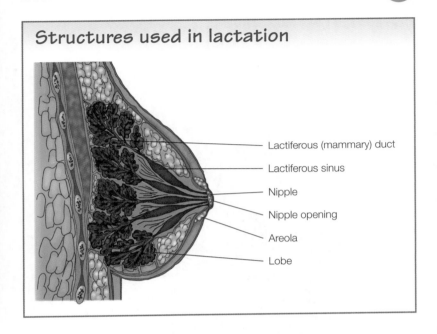

Lactiferous (mammary) duct

Lactiferous sinus

Nipple

Nipple opening

Areola

Lobe

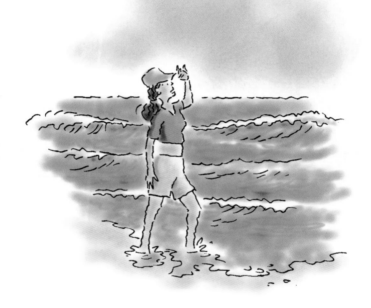

Anatomy & Physiology Made Incredibly Easy, 3rd ed. Philadelphia: Lippincott Williams & Wilkins, 2009.

Anatomy & Physiology Made Incredibly Visual. Philadelphia: Lippincott Williams & Wilkins, 2008.

Bianchi, J., and Cameron, J. "Assessment of Skin Integrity in the Elderly," *British Journal of Community Nursing* 13(3):S26, S28, S30-2, March 2008.

Chirico, G., et al. "Anti-infective Properties of Human Milk," *Journal of Nutrition* 138(9):1801S-06S, September 2008.

Eken, C. "Acidosis Is a Life-threatening Condition Regardless of the Underlying Condition," *American Journal of Emergency Medicine* 26(6):721, July 2008.

Elia, M., and Cummings, J.H. "Physiological Aspects of Energy Metabolism and Gastrointestinal Effects of Carbohydrates," *European Journal of Clinical Nutrition* 61(Suppl. 1):S40-74, December 2007.

Ersser, S.J., et al. "Research Activity and Evidence-based Practice within DNA: A Survey," *Dermatology Nursing* 20(3):189-94, June 2008.

Hill, K.M. "Surgical Repair of Cardiac Valves," *Critical Care Nursing Clinics of North America* 19(4):353-60, December 2007.

Jones, E.Y., et al. "T Cell Receptors Get Back to Basics," *Nature Immunology* 8(10):1033-35, October 2007.

Roberts, M.M. "Neurophysiology in Neurourology," *Muscle & Nerve* 38(1):815-36, July 2008.

Saladin, K.S. *Anatomy and Physiology: The Unity of Form and Function, 4th ed.* New York: McGraw-Hill, 2007.

Scanlon, V.C., et al. *Essentials of Anatomy and Physiology, 5th ed.* Philadelphia: F.A. Davis, 2007.

Sitzman, K. "The New Food Pyramid," *AAOHN Journal* 54(1):48, January 2006.

Smeltzer, S.C., et al. *Brunner and Suddarth's Textbook of Medical-Surgical Nursing, 11th ed.* Philadelphia: Lippincott Williams & Wilkins, 2008.

Straight A's in Anatomy and Physiology. Philadelphia: Lippincott Williams & Wilkins, 2007.

Sullivan, M.C., et al. "Developmental Origins Theory from Prematurity to Adult Disease," *Journal of Obstetrics, Gynecologic, and Neonatal Nursing* 37(2):158-64, March-April 2008.

Note: t refers to a table; i refers to an illustration.

Note: t refers to a table; i refers to an illustration.

Note: t refers to a table; i refers to an illustration.

Note: t refers to a table; i refers to an illustration.

Note: t refers to a table; i refers to an illustration.

Note: t refers to a table; i refers to an illustration.

Note: t refers to a table; i refers to an illustration.

Note: t refers to a table; i refers to an illustration.